A Million Person Household Survey: Understanding the Burden of Injuries in Bangladesh

Special Issue Editors

Adnan A. Hyder
Olakunle Alonge

MDPI • Basel • Beijing • Wuhan • Barcelona • Belgrade

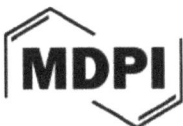

MDPI

Special Issue Editors
Adnan A. Hyder
Johns Hopkins University
USA

Olakunle Alonge
Johns Hopkins University
USA

Editorial Office
MDPI
St. Alban-Anlage 66
Basel, Switzerland

This edition is a reprint of the Special Issue published online in the open access journal *International Journal of Environmental Research and Public Health* (ISSN 1660-4601) from 2017–2018 (available at: http://www.mdpi.com/journal/ijerph/special issues/Injuries Bangladesh).

For citation purposes, cite each article independently as indicated on the article page online and as indicated below:

Lastname, F.M.; Lastname, F.M. Article title. *Journal Name* **Year**, *Article number*, page range.

First Editon 2018

Cover image courtesy of Kuni Takahashi

ISBN 978-3-03842-969-2 (Pbk)
ISBN 978-3-03842-970-8 (PDF)

Table of Contents

About the Special Issue Editors

Adnan A. Hyder, professor and associate chair of the Department of International Health; director of the Health Systems Program and Johns Hopkins International Injury Research Unit at the Johns Hopkins Bloomberg School of Public Health in USA has 20 years of global health experience in low- and middle-income countries. Dr. Hyder leads a team of experts to conduct groundbreaking research on health systems strengthening and capacity building. Dr. Hyder is well known for his work on health systems analysis and health decisions; for developing the healthy life year indicator; and for exploring the research to policy interface in health systems in developing countries. Dr. Hyder has co-authored more than 300 scientific papers and world reports on topics such as health systems, biomedical ethics, and road traffic and child injuries. Dr. Hyder did his MD from the Aga Khan University, Pakistan and obtained his MPH and PhD in Public Health from Johns Hopkins University, USA.

Olakunle Alonge, MD PhD MPH is an Assistant Professor in the Department of International Health at the Bloomberg School of Public Health, Johns Hopkins University (JHSPH). Dr. Alonge obtained his medical degree from the University of Ibadan in Nigeria, and was subsequently trained in epidemiology and biostatistics at the Johns Hopkins University. He obtained is PhD also from the Johns Hopkins University with a focus on international health systems. Dr. Alonge's current research at the JHSPH is focused on implementation science as applicable to addressing the burden of injuries, strengthening health systems and closing health inequities gaps in low and middle-income countries (LMICs). Prior to joining JHSPH, Dr. Alonge managed the provision of primary health services in Nigeria and Liberia, and assessed health systems performance, provided monitoring and evaluation services for technical assistance in strengthening health activities and research in Afghanistan. At JHSPH, Dr. Alonge managed the Johns Hopkins International Injury Research Unit (JH-IIRU's) program in Bangladesh on child drowning, and worked on measuring and quantifying the burden of injuries and effect of drowning prevention interventions in Bangladesh, Uganda and Vietnam. He has also worked in understanding the epidemiology of child injuries, and level of policy response to this burden in Ethiopia. In collaboration with the WHO, he developed a framework for assessing child injury policies at global and national level, and tracking progress in primary prevention of various mechanisms of child injuries in LMICs. Currently, Dr. Alonge works on implementing social accountability interventions for strengthening health systems in Bangladesh and Uganda, and understanding factors contributing to health systems resilience in Liberia. He is also the PI for an implementation science grant on lessons learned from the Global Polio Eradication Initiative (GPEI) involving a consortium of academic partners from seven LMICs (Nigeria, Democratic Republic of Congo, Ethiopia, Afghanistan, Bangladesh, India and Indonesia). He provides implementation science support for school-based mental health programs for the WHO Eastern Mediterranean region. At JHSPH, Dr. Alonge teaches courses on implementation research and practices, health equity and social justice, and confronting the burden of injuries; and provides mentorship and service for students in the Health Systems Program at the school. Dr. Alonge is also the co-director for the JHSPH Doctorate in Public Health program, Health Equity and Social Justice concentration. Read more about his work in his faculty profile.

International Journal of
*Environmental Research
and Public Health*

MDPI

Editorial

Burden of Injuries in Bangladesh:
A Population-Based Assessment

Priyanka Agrawaland Adnan A. Hyder *

Department of International Health, International Injury Research Unit, Johns Hopkins University Bloomberg School of Public Health, Baltimore, MD 21205, USA; pagrawa6@jhu.edu
* Correspondence: ahyder1@jhu.edu

Received: 13 February 2018; Accepted: 23 February 2018; Published: 27 February 2018

Keywords: injury; population-based; survey; drowning; epidemiology; Bangladesh

Injuries claim over 5 million lives, with more than 90% of those occurring in low- and middle-income countries (LMICS) [1,2]. Unintentional injuries such as drowning, road traffic injuries, falls and burns account for 72% of all injury deaths. Drowning, one of the leading causes of unintentional injuries across the world, accounted for more than 300,000 deaths in 2016 [3]. This collection documents some of the epidemiological findings on the burden of injuries, both intentional and unintentional, in Bangladesh, in the context of a large, multi-year, population-based project—Saving of Lives from Drowning (SoLiD).

SoLiD was established with the main objective of evaluating the large-scale effectiveness and value for money of interventions—crèches and playpens—in the reduction of drowning mortality and morbidity in children less than 5 years of age. The project conducted a baseline census in seven rural sub-districts of Bangladesh and covered over 1.2 million individuals, in order to collect demographic and injury-related information. An injury surveillance system was set up to collect injury outcomes on a quarterly basis for 3 years, and compliance assessments on a monthly basis to test the usability and acceptability of the interventions.

This collection highlights the epidemiology and risk factors for injuries prevalent in rural Bangladesh, and showcases the depth of information generated from a large population-based survey. While the collection provides a snapshot of the burden of injury in a low- and middle-income country such as Bangladesh, it also highlights the slow progress, via the dearth of available evidence-based effective interventions, programs and policies present to address this burden.

In Bangladesh, while childhood deaths due to communicable infectious diseases were on a decline in the past decade, deaths due to injuries in the same age group were increasing. The paper *Epidemiology of Drowning in Bangladesh: An Update* shows that children 1 to 5 years of age were 13 to 16 times more likely to be involved in a drowning (or near-drowning) event than infants or older children. Individuals from lower socio-economic profiles were at more risk of drowning than their rich counterparts. Males also sustained more near-drowning events than females.

A similar gender trend is highlighted in the paper on the *Pattern of Road Traffic Injuries in Rural Bangladesh: Burden Estimates and Risk Factors*. The authors suggest developing policies and programs to make pedestrian-friendly road networks and reinforcement of helmet use, given that pedestrians and two-wheel drivers sustained more than one-third of road traffic injuries.

In contrast, burn injuries and suicides were three to six times more common in females than in males in the rural population of Bangladesh. In *Epidemiology of Burns in Rural Bangladesh: An Update*, the authors also overcame the issue of under-reporting and underestimation of the burden of burn injuries in a LMIC setting. In *The Burden of Suicide in Rural Bangladesh: Magnitude and Risk Factors*, adolescent girls and young married women, aged 15 to 24 years of age, showcased a very specific age group at a disproportionately high risk.

Additionally, in *Epidemiology of Fall Injury in Rural Bangladesh*, elderly people, 65 years of age and above, were seen to be at highest risk of both fatal and non-fatal fall injuries. The physical, mental and emotional wellbeing of elderly individuals can be disrupted by a debilitating fall injury and drive them into greater vulnerability. These papers highlight the need for targeted approaches in the form of interventions, policy changes and programs to address respective burdens of disease.

The notion of a center-based, early childhood education program may not be entirely new in Bangladesh, but there is a lack of research on the cognitive benefits of such an approach in LMICs. In high-income countries, it has been shown that early childhood education has both short term and long-term benefits for children exposed to it. The paper *Developmental Assessments during Injury Research: Is Enrollment of Very Young Children in Crèches Associated with Better Scores?* showed that being enrolled in a crèche intervention had a positive dose-response relationship on fine and gross motor skills, personal–social and problem-solving skills for children 1–5 years of age. This reiterated the importance of engaging young children in formal age-appropriate education systems.

The authors of *Caregiver Supervision Practices and Risk of Childhood Unintentional Injury Mortality in Bangladesh*, used a large population-level dataset to suggest that adult caregiver supervision significantly reduced the risk of drowning deaths for children under 5 years of age. This notion of adult supervision needs to be effectively communicated amongst communities in LMICs, mainly because injuries are still conceived of as unforeseeable "accidents" that cannot be prevented. Additionally, with injuries comes a high risk of sustaining a long-term disability, along with loss of productivity and other economic costs. First aid, by a formal medical provider, can improve the odds of faster recovery for an individual with injuries. However, informal providers are readily available in LMICs such as Bangladesh. Thus, authors of the paper *Impact of First Aid on Treatment Outcomes for Non-Fatal Injuries in Rural Bangladesh: Findings from an Injury and Demographic Census*, suggest that public health interventions should be designed to train and improve first aid skills for informal providers.

It is important to consider the economic ramifications of injuries and associated disabilities, because the majority one-income households in rural Bangladesh undergo financial distress in dealing with the aftermath of fatal and non-fatal injuries. In the paper, *Care-Seeking Patterns and Direct Economic Burden of Injuries in Bangladesh*, the authors tested the relationship between care-seeking behavior of injured households and financial distress, and suggested that enforcing occupational safety regulations, worksite inspections, home safety inspections and such promotions, should help alleviate the economic distress caused by injury.

This collection of papers, therefore, provides a base for new channels of future research. These scholars have shown correlations between injury and age, sex and wealth. Additionally, they focus on demonstrating the link between various types of interventions—be it childcare centers, playpens, or first aid training—and injury prevention. What needs further study is *why* certain correlations exist and the *how* specific interventions work. To address these deficiencies, future studies must be of longer duration to include the eventual impact and include qualitative measurements of behavior to trace links between risks and actual injury prevention. The group involved in these papers is now working to address this gap in incidence. When researchers have a better handle on causal links, they can also look at antecedents, such as cultural and social norms, that influence behavior, all questions that need to be addressed to reduce the millions of deaths caused by injuries around the world.

Author Contributions: A.A.H. is the guarantor of the project and participated in the design, implementation and supervision of the project as well as reviewed and edited the manuscript. P.A. conceptualized the idea for the manuscript, wrote the initial and subsequent drafts of the manuscript.

Conflicts of Interest: The authors declare no conflict of interest. The funding sponsors had no role in the design of the study; in the collection, analyses, or interpretation of data; in the writing of the manuscript, and in the decision to publish the results.

Int. J. Environ. Res. Public Health **2018**, *15*, 409

References

1. World Health Organization. *The Injury Chart Book: A Graphical Overview of the Global Burden of Injuries;* World Health Organization: Geneva, Switzerland, 2002.
2. World Health Organization. *Injuries and Violence: the Facts 2014;* World Health Organization: Geneva, Switzerland, 2014.
3. Global Health Data Exchange. Institute for Health Metrics and Evaluation. Available online: http://ghdx.healthdata.org/gbd-results-tool (accessed on 13 February 2018).

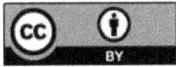

International Journal of
*Environmental Research
and Public Health*

MDPI

Article

Epidemiology of Drowning in Bangladesh: An Update

Aminur Rahman [1,*], Olakunle Alonge [2], Al-Amin Bhuiyan [1], Priyanka Agrawal [2], Shumona Sharmin Salam [3], Abu Talab [1], Qazi Sadeq-ur Rahman [3] and Adnan A. Hyder [2]

[1] Centre for Injury Prevention and Research, Bangladesh (CIPRB), House B162, Road 23, New DOHS, Mohakhali, Dhaka 1206, Bangladesh; al-amin@ciprb.org (A.-A.B.); abutalab01@ciprb.org (A.T.)
[2] Johns Hopkins International Injury Research Unit, Department of International Health, Johns Hopkins Bloomberg School of Public Health, 615 N. Wolfe Street, Baltimore, MD 21205, USA; oalonge1@jhu.edu (O.A.); pagrawa6@jhu.edu (P.A.); ahyder1@jhu.edu (A.A.H.)
[3] Centre for Child and Adolescent Health, icddr,b. 68 Shaheed Tajuddin Ahmed Sarani, Mohakhali, Dhaka 1212, Bangladesh; shumona@icddrb.org (S.S.S.); qsrahman@icddrb.org (Q.S.R.)
* Correspondence: aminur@ciprb.org; Tel.: +880-171-512-809

Academic Editor: David C. Schwebel
Received: 22 February 2017; Accepted: 3 May 2017; Published: 5 May 2017

Abstract: Over one-quarter of deaths among 1–4 year-olds in Bangladesh were due to drowning in 2003, and the proportion increased to 42% in 2011. This study describes the current burden and risk factors for drowning across all demographics in rural Bangladesh. A household survey was carried out in 51 union parishads of rural Bangladesh between June and November 2013, covering 1.17 million individuals. Information on fatal and nonfatal drowning events was collected by face-to-face interviews using a structured questionnaire. Fatal and non-fatal drowning rates were 15.8/100,000/year and 318.4/100,000/6 months, respectively, for all age groups. The highest rates of fatal (121.5/100,000/year) and non-fatal (3057.7/100,000/6 months) drowning were observed among children 1 to 4 years of age. These children had higher rates of fatal (13 times) and non-fatal drowning (16 times) compared with infants. Males had slightly higher rates of both fatal and non-fatal drowning. Individuals with no education had 3 times higher rates of non-fatal drowning compared with those with high school or higher education. Non-fatal drowning rates increased significantly with decrease in socio-economic status (SES) quintiles, from the highest to the lowest. Drowning is a major public health issue in Bangladesh, and is now a major threat to child survival.

Keywords: drowning rate; fatal; non-fatal; rural areas; risk-factors; Bangladesh

1. Introduction

The World Health Organization (WHO) estimated that 372,000 deaths occurred from drowning in 2012, which has made it the world's third leading unintentional injury killer [1]. Over half of all drowning deaths occur among those under 25 years of age. Ninety-one percent of drowning deaths across all ages occur in low- and middle-income countries (LMICs) [2]. Fatal drowning rates among children in LMICs are 6 times higher than that of high-income countries (HICs), and several studies suggest that children aged 1–4 years are at the highest risk [3–8].

The Bangladesh Health and Injury Survey (BHIS) conducted in 2003–2004 revealed that drowning was the leading cause of deaths in children 1–17 years of age (28.6 per 100,000 children-years), and children 1–4 years-old were at highest risk (86.3 per 100,000 children-years) of drowning. The study also showed that the proportion of all deaths due to drowning among 1–4 year-olds was 26.0% in 2005; by 2011 this had increased to 42.0% [9,10].

In the HICs, drowning often occurs in recreational swimming pools [11–13], whereas in LMICs drowning happens in natural water bodies such as ponds, ditches, rivers, lakes, and dams [14–16]. Risk factors for childhood drowning in LMICs include, but are not limited to, inadequate supervision, male sex, lack of physical barriers between people and water bodies, and lack of swimming ability [8,16–18]. Lack of water safety awareness, risky behavior around water, and perceived risk are also considered important risk factors [19–21]. Travelling on overcrowded or poorly maintained vessels and water related disasters (e.g., flood, extreme rainfall, storm surges, and tsunamis or cyclones) are also common risk factors in all age groups globally [2].

Two supervisory tools, door barriers and playpens, were piloted in rural areas of Bangladesh, in an attempt to reduce drowning [17,18]. The findings suggested that both tools improved supervision; however, caregivers preferred playpens [18]. Another study explored the option of community crèches and reported that children who participated in the crèche program were 80% less likely to drown than those who did not participate [18,22].

However, as no nationwide childhood drowning prevention program has been implemented in Bangladesh, drowning continues to be the leading cause of death among children 1–4 years of age. Drowning also remains a leading cause of injury deaths among all age groups [23]. These estimates are based on modeled data and there is a lack of population-based data to describe the epidemiology, magnitude, and risk factors for drowning across all ages, and more specifically in children in Bangladesh. Such knowledge would be important for designing and implementing drowning prevention strategies that are responsive to the current risk factors not only in Bangladesh, but also in other LMICs with similar contexts.

The objective of this study was to describe the burden and risk factors of drowning for all demographics in rural Bangladesh, including children 1–4 years-old using data from a population-based census conducted in 2013. This paper aims to fill the gap in knowledge about the burden of drowning among all populations and provide updates on risk factors for drowning in rural Bangladesh.

2. Methods

A large-scale implementation project "Saving of Lives from Drowning" (SoLiD) was conducted in Bangladesh to test the effectiveness of childhood drowning prevention interventions. As part of the project, a baseline census was conducted between June and November of 2013 in 51 union parishads of seven rural sub-districts of Bangladesh: Matlab North, Matlab South, Daudkandi, Chandpur Sadar, Raiganj, Sherpur Sadar, and Manohardi. The census covered 1.17 million population and 270,387 households in these 51 union parishads.

Trained data collectors used pre-tested structured questionnaires to collect information from household heads or any adult above 18 years by face-to-face interviews. Data collection occurred in two stages. In the first stage, demographic, socio-economic, illness, and health-seeking information was collected for all members of the household. Household members who had any injury event were also identified during the first stage. In the second stage, information on injury morbidity and mortality were collected for both intentional and unintentional injuries. Injury was operationally defined as any external harm resulting from any assault, fall, cut, burn, animal bite, poisoning, transportation, operation of machinery, blunt objects, suffocation, or drowning related event resulting in the loss of one or more days of normal daily activities, school, or work. Drowning was described as the process of experiencing respiratory impairment from submersion or immersion in liquid [24]. Non-fatal drowning was operationally defined as survival from a drowning event. Information on all fatal injuries was collected over a one-year recall period, and over a six-month recall period for non-fatal injuries.

To ensure the quality of data, trained supervisors were recruited, and they observed 10% of interviews conducted by the data collectors, checked 10% of the collected data, and re-interviewed 2% of the households. In addition, field level research officers and managers were appointed to re-check all data for inconsistencies. If any inconsistency was found, the respective data collector was asked to revisit the household to collect correct information.

Ethical clearance for this study was obtained from the Institutional Review Boards of the Johns Hopkins Bloomberg School of Public Health in the USA, the Center for Injury Prevention Research, Bangladesh, and the International Centre for Diarrheal Disease Research, Bangladesh.

All records of fatal and non-fatal drowning were retrieved from the primary database for the current analysis. A description of the population by fatal and non-fatal drowning, sex, age, level of education, socio-economic status (SES) (computed based on a principal component analysis of household asset variables), and sub-districts was provided with proportion. Frequency distribution and proportion of different variables related to fatal and non-fatal drowning were also calculated. The descriptor variables included place of drowning, distance of water bodies from home, time of occurrence, and the seasonality of drowning. Drowning rates were calculated per 100,000 populations per year for fatal drowning and per 100,000 populations per 6 months for non-fatal drowning. These rates were further disaggregated by age, sex, SES, education, and sub-district levels. Fatal and non-fatal drowning outcomes were modeled as odds ratios comparing levels of independent variables such as age, sex, SES, and education using logistic regressions. Results from both bivariate and multivariate analyses are presented.

3. Results

The census covered 1.17 million people from seven selected sub-districts of Bangladesh. The proportion of females (51.5%) was slightly higher than males (48.5%). Among the total population, 9.6% were children under five years of age, 29.4% were 5 to 17 years of age, and about 61% were adults (18 years and over). Over one-quarter (25.3%) of the population had no formal education, however, about 60.0% had either primary or secondary level education. Considering the SES index, the population was divided into quintiles and the proportion of population in each category of SES index was almost the same, ranging between 18.1% and 21.6%. The proportion of the population in each sub-district varied depending upon the number of union parishads covered from the selected sub-district for the census (Table 1).

Table 1. Description of population by sex, age, level of education, socio-economic status (SES) index, sub-districts, and fatal and non-fatal drowning outcomes.

Characteristics	Counts (N)	Frequency (%)
Sex		
Male	567,674	48.54
Female	601,919	51.46
Age Group		
<1 year	22,141	1.89
1–4 years	90,523	7.74
5–9 years	139,728	11.95
10–14 years	142,121	12.15
15–17 years	62,098	5.31
18–24 years	133,534	11.42
25–64 years	508,059	43.44
65+ years	71,389	6.10
Level of Education		
No education	295,314	25.3
Primary	407,923	34.9
Secondary	289,658	24.8
A levels and above	63,873	5.5
Not applicable (<5 years)	112,664	9.6

Table 1. *Cont.*

Characteristics	Counts (N)	Frequency (%)
Socio-Economic Index		
Lowest	211,610	18.1
Low	218,695	18.7
Middle	238,371	20.4
High	247,716	21.2
Highest	253,210	21.6
Sub-Districts		
Matlab North	265,897	22.7
Matlab South	209,772	17.9
Chandpur Sadar	128,356	11.0
Raiganj	104,357	8.9
Sherpur Sadar	228,519	19.5
Manohardi	204,319	17.5
Daudkandi	28,373	2.4
Drowning		
Fatal (1 year recall)	185	0.016
Non-fatal (6 months recall)	3752	0.321

One hundred eighty-five fatal drowning cases in the year preceding the census and 3752 non-fatal drowning events in the preceding six months of the census were identified (Table 1). Among the non-fatal drowning cases, about 19.0% had multiple events. All cases of fatal drowning were unintentional in nature.

Fatal and non-fatal drowning rates were 15.8/100,000 per year and 318.4/100,000 per 6 months, respectively. Both fatal and non-fatal drowning rates were found higher among males (fatal: 19.0/100,000 per year; 95% confidence interval (95% CI) 15.7–23.1 and non-fatal: 372.6/100,000 per 6 months; 95% CI 357.1–388.8) than females (fatal: 12.8/100,000 per year; 95% CI 10.2–16.1 and non-fatal: 267.1/(254.3–280.5)). The difference of rates between male and female in non-fatal drowning was statistically significant.

The highest rates of fatal and non-fatal drowning were observed in children 1–4 years of age at 121.5/100,000 per year (95% CI 100.3–147.0) and 3057.7/100,000 in 6 months (95% CI 2948.0–3172.0), respectively. Among adults (18 years and over), the highest rate (8.4/100,000 per year; 95% CI 3.4–19.3) of fatal drowning was found among the 65 years and older age group; and the highest non-fatal drowning rates (28.4/100,000 per 6 months; 95% CI 24.1–33.49) were found among 25–64 year-olds.

Higher rates of fatal (12.5/100,000 per year; 95% CI 8.9–17.5) and non-fatal drowning (139.6/100,000 per 6 months; 95% CI 126.4–153.6) were observed among those who did not have any education compared to the educated groups.

The highest rates for both fatal (21.7/100,000 per year; 16.1–29.3) and non-fatal drowning (504.1/100,000; 474.7–535.3) were observed in the most deprived SES quintile, and with the increase of SES index the incidence rates decreased. However, the fatal drowning incidence rate was found to be slightly higher (13.0/100,000 per year) in the wealthiest quintile (highest) than the wealthy quintile (high) (11.3/100,000 per year).

Fatal drowning rates were found to be similar in all sub-districts, ranging from 16.7 to 20.3/100,000 per year, except in Sherpur Sadar (12.3/100,000 population per year) and Manohardi (12.2/100,000 population per year). The highest fatal drowning rate was observed in Chandpur Sadar (20.3/100,000 population per year) and the lowest in Manohardi (Table 2). Significant variations were found in comparisons of non-fatal drowning rates between sub-districts (Table 2), with the highest non-fatal drowning rates in Raiganj, followed by Daudkandi, Matlab South, and Matlab North.

Table 2. Fatal and non-fatal drowning rates (per 100,000) by sex, age, level of education, SES index, and sub-districts.

Variables	Fatal Drowning		Non-Fatal Drowning	
	Population (N)	Rate/100,000/ Year (95% CI)	Population (N)	Rate/100,000/6 Months (95% CI)
Sex				
Both	1,169,593	15.8 (13.6–18.3)	1,178,256	318.4 (308.4–328.8)
Male	567,674	19.0 (15.7–23.1)	573,225	372.6 (357.1–388.8)
Female	601,919	12.8 (10.2–16.1)	605,031	267.1 (254.3–280.5)
Age in Years				
<1 year	22,141	9.0 (1.6–36.4)	21,594	171.3 (122.4–234.7)
1–4 years	90,523	121.5 (100.3–147.0)	91,737	3057.7 (2948.0–3172.0)
5–9 years	139,728	22.9 (15.9–32.7)	141,024	465.9 (428.3–499.6)
10–14 years	142,121	5.6 (2.6–11.6)	143,206	37.0 (28.0–48.8)
15–17 years	62,098	3.2 (0.6–13.0)	62,580	14.4 (7.0–28.38)
18–24 years	133,534	6.7 (3.3–13.3)	134,535	19.3 (12.9–28.76)
25–64 years	508,059	3.1 (1.9–5.2)	514,264	28.4 (24.1–33.49)
65+ years	71,389	8.4 (3.4–19.3)	69,316	27.4 (17.0–43.69)
Level of Education				
No education	295,314	12.5 (8.9–17.5)	296,357	139.6 (126.4–153.6)
Primary	407,923	6.9 (4.6–10.1)	412,140	108.8 (98.1–118.3)
Secondary	289,658	1.7 (0.6–4.3)	292,118	15.9 (11.7–21.2)
Higher secondary level and above	63,873	3.1 (0.5–12.6)	64,158	10.9 (4.8–23.6)
Not applicable (<5 children)	112,664	100.3 (83.0–121.0)	113,331	2522.5 (2418.0–2601.0)
SES Index				
Lowest	211,601	21.7 (16.1–29.3)	213,242	504.1 (474.7–535.3)
Low	218,695	18.7 (13.6–25.7)	220,666	375.2 (350.3–401.8)
Middle	238,371	15.5 (11.1–21.6)	240,313	297.5 (276.3–320.3)
High	247,716	11.3 (7.7–16.6)	249,546	253.3 (234.1–274.0)
Highest	253,210	13.0 (9.1–18.5)	254,489	197.3 (180.6–215.5)
Sub-District				
Matlab North	265,897	17.3 (12.8–23.3)	267,748	306.5 (284.0–326.2)
Matlab South	209,772	16.7 (11.8–23.5)	213,691	531.5 (491.9–553.5)
Chandpur Sadar	128,356	20.3 (13.5–30.1)	128,671	194.0 (170.6–219.5)
Raiganj	104,357	19.2 (12.0–30.2)	106,044	885.4 (816.7–929.6)
Sherpur Sadar	228,519	12.3 (8.3–18.0)	228,591	107.6 (94.78–122.2)
Manohardi	204,319	12.2 (8.1–18.4)	204,551	113.5 (99.51–129.2)
Daudkandi	28,373	17.6 (6.5–43.7)	28,960	602.7 (507.0–687.3)

CI: Confidence Interval.

Multiple logistic regression analysis showed that males were at higher risk of both fatal and non-fatal drowning than females. Children 1–4 years of age were 13.3 times (CI 3.3–54.0; $p = 0.000$) and 15.9 times (CI 11.2–22.5; $p = 0.000$) higher at risk of fatal and non-fatal drowning, respectively, than infants (<1 year). Although individuals in other older age groups were also at higher risk of fatal drowning, the odds ratios were not statistically significant. In the case of non-fatal drowning, the analysis showed a statistically significant higher risk in all age groups compared to infants. Individuals with no education had 3.7 times (CI 0.8–16.7; $p = 0.1$) and about 2.9 times (CI 1.3–6.7; $p = 0.013$) higher risk of fatal and non-fatal drowning, respectively, than those who had secondary level education or higher. With the decrease of SES quintile from the highest to the lowest, the risk of fatal and non-fatal drowning increased; this association was, however, only significant for non-fatal drowning events (Table 3).

Table 3. Association between socio-demographic factors and drowning events, fatal and non-fatal.

Characteristics	Fatal Drowning				Non-Fatal Drowning			
	OR (95% CI) Unadjusted	p Value	OR (95% CI) Adjusted	p Value	OR (95% CI) Unadjusted	p Value	OR (95% CI) Adjusted	p Value
Sex								
Male	1.5 (1.1–2.0)	0.008	1.4 (1.0–1.9)	0.030	1.4 (1.3–1.5)	0.000	1.2 (1.1–1.3)	0.000
Female	1		1		1		1	
Age Groups (Years)								
<1 year	1		1		1		1	
1–4 years	13.5 (3.3–54.5)	0.000	13.3 (3.3–54.0)	0.000	18.4 (13.3–25.4)	0.000	15.9 (11.2–22.5)	0.000
5–9 years	2.5 (0.6–10.6)	0.20	1.3 (0.2–10.1)	0.818	2.7 (2.0–3.8)	0.000	1.5 (0.6–3.6)	0.423
10–14 years	0.6 (0.1–2.9)	0.56	0.5 (0.1–4.4)	0.537	0.2 (0.1–0.3)	0.000	0.2 (0.1–0.4)	0.000
15–17 years	0.4 (0.1–2.5)	0.30	0.4 (0.0–4.2)	0.428	0.1 (0.04–0.17)	0.000	0.1 (0.0–0.2)	0.000
18–24 years	0.8 (0.2–3.5)	0.71	0.7 (0.1–4.7)	0.673	0.11 (0.07–0.19)	0.000	0.1 (0.0–0.2)	0.000
25–64 years	0.4 (0.1–1.5)	0.16	0.2 (0.0–1.3)	0.084	0.67 (0.12–0.24)	0.000	0.1 (0.0–0.2)	0.000
65+ years	0.9 (0.2–4.6)	0.93	0.3 (0.0–3.0)	0.323	0.16 (0.09–0.28)	0.000	0.1 (0.0–0.2)	0.000
Level of Education								
No education	4.0 (1.0–16.6)	0.05	3.7 (0.8–16.7)	0.100	12.8 (6.1–27.0)	0.000	2.9 (1.3–6.7)	0.013
Primary	2.2 (0.5–9.2)	0.28	1.3 (0.3–6.1)	0.728	9.9 (4.7–20.9)	0.000	1.4 (0.6–3.1)	0.480
Secondary	0.6 (0.1–2.8)	0.47	0.6 (0.1–3.0)	0.506	1.4 (0.7–3.2)	0.37	1.1 (0.5–2.7)	0.776
A levels and above	1		1		1		1	
SES Index								
Lowest	1.7 (1.1–2.6)	0.02	1.3 (0.8–2.1)	0.234	2.6 (2.3–2.9)	0.000	2.0 (1.8–2.3)	0.000
Low	1.4 (0.9–2.3)	0.12	1.3 (0.8–2.1)	0.250	1.9 (1.7–2.1)	0.000	1.8 (1.6–2.1)	0.000
Middle	1.2 (0.7–1.9)	0.46	1.1 (0.7–1.8)	0.656	1.5 (1.4–1.7)	0.000	1.4 (1.3–1.6)	0.000
High	0.9 (0.5–1.4)	0.57	0.8 (0.5–1.4)	0.500	1.3 (1.1–1.5)	0.000	1.4 (1.2–1.6)	0.000
Highest	1		1		1		1	

OR: Odds Ratio.

9

Natural bodies of water such as ponds, ditches, lakes, and rivers were common places of drowning. Ponds were the most common place (66.0%) of drowning in Bangladesh. About three-quarters (73.0%) of drowning took place in bodies of water within 20 m from the victims' house. Almost all (95.0%) drowning occurred during the daylight between 0900 h and 1800 h, of which almost two-thirds occurred before 1300 h. The study revealed a seasonal pattern of drowning which showed an increase of drowning during monsoon, with peaks in July and the winters (November–January) relatively free of drowning events (Figure 1).

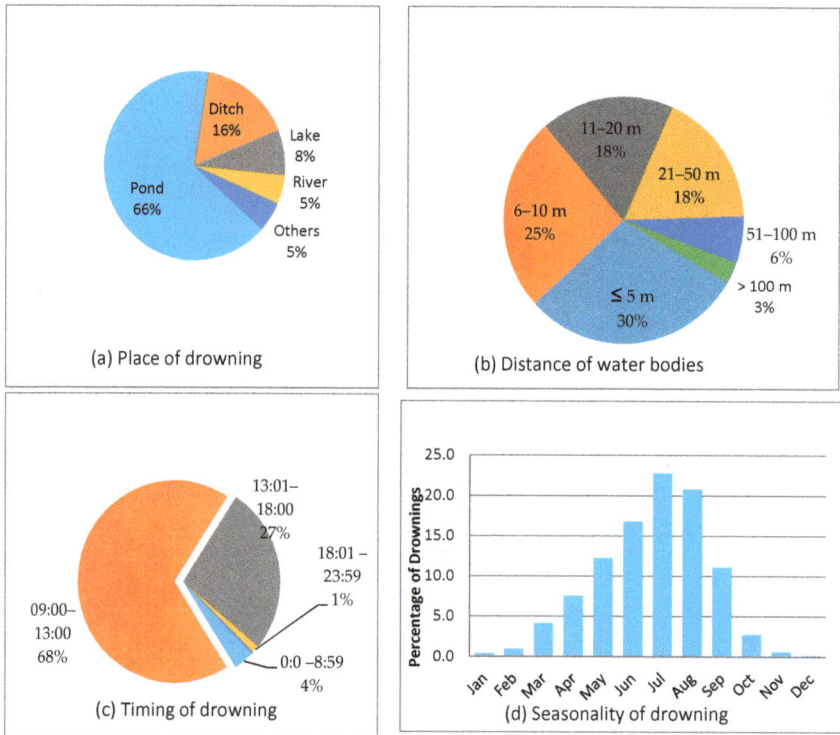

Figure 1. Factors associated with fatal and non-fatal drowning: (**a**) Place of drowning; (**b**) Distance of water bodies; (**c**) Timing of drowning; (**d**) Seasonality of drowning.

4. Discussion

As in other LMICs, the reporting system for deaths and health related events is weak in Bangladesh. Thus, it is very difficult to ascertain the burden of diseases and injuries in the country based on routinely collected data. In addition, most recent population-based research on the burden of drowning in the country is quite dated [25–28]. Therefore, this study, using recent population-based data, provides a comprehensive update on the burden and epidemiology of drowning in Bangladesh. In this survey, household visits were conducted to collect relevant data on fatal and non-fatal drowning events for over 1 million people.

This study suggests that across all ages, the fatal drowning rate was 15.8 per 100,000 people per year and the non-fatal drowning rate was 318.4 per 100,000 per 6 months in rural Bangladesh. According to the WHO Global Report on Drowning, rates of drowning in LMICs, such as Bangladesh, are higher than in HICs, and in comparing LMICs, the fatal drowning rate in Bangladesh is 2 to 5 times higher than rates from most other LMICs based on the 2012 WHO Global Health Estimates [1,2].

These findings suggest that the burden of global drowning may be disproportionately borne by a few LMICs, including Bangladesh; thus, initial efforts on global drowning prevention may focus on such countries.

Within Bangladesh, while no variations were noticed in the fatal drowning rates, significant variations were observed in non-fatal drowning rates comparing geographical regions in the seven Upazilas surveyed in rural Bangladesh, and sub-districts such as Raiganj, Daudkandi, Matlab North and Matlab South had significantly higher rates. These differences in the non-fatal drowning relative to drowning rates may be indicative of the differences in the level of awareness about the risk of drowning, exposure to water bodies, and coverage of drowning prevention activities between these sub-districts. For instance, Raiganj was seen to have the highest fatal and non-fatal drowning events, in spite of having SwimSafe programs and crèches in their communities for over a decade [26]. It is probable that due to awareness among residents in the community about injury prevention programs, there were higher self-reporting instances. In addition, Matlab North, Matlab South, Chandpur Sadar, and Daudkandi have more natural water bodies in and around them, which when considered along with all other risk factors, puts its residents at a higher risk of drowning events.

The rates for both fatal and non-fatal drowning were higher among males when compared to females, which is similar to other LMICs, as reported by the WHO Global Report on Drowning [2]. The higher risk among males can probably be attributed to higher exposure to risky situations, increased risk taking behavior, and involvement in activities outside the home among males [27].

The highest rates of fatal and non-fatal drowning were observed in children 1–4 years of age followed by 5–9 year-olds children. These findings are similar to findings from a previously conducted national survey, Bangladesh Health and Injury Survey (BHIS) 2005, and reflect the trend that rural children aged 1–4 years are the worst affected by drowning in Bangladesh, and that this trend has not changed over the past decade [2,8]. Similar findings have also been reported in other East-Asian countries such as Thailand, Vietnam, and China [28], and countries in the Western Pacific Region [29]. The increased risk of drowning among children under five years of age has been associated with lack of adequate adult supervision, combined with environmental risks, and behavioral factors such as increased curiosity among toddlers, lack of ample dexterity and co-ordination, and limited cognitive awareness of their surroundings [2,15,26].

Low educational level and poor socio-economic status were associated with higher drowning rates for both fatal and non-fatal events, and similar findings have also been reported in previous studies from Bangladesh [30–32]. Such disparities in drowning outcomes may suggest disproportionate access to safe environments, knowledge around drowning prevention, and relevant rescue and health services when comparing populations of different socioeconomic status. Thus, these results highlight the need for prioritizing populations from low socioeconomic status backgrounds in drowning prevention efforts.

In this study, most drowning events occurred in ponds and ditches, almost all located within 20 m from the residences of victims, and most frequently during the annual monsoon season, similar to findings reported in prior studies [15,22,28]. Given the tropical climate in Bangladesh, monsoon rainfalls may lead to floods, and increased water levels in rivers, canals, ponds, and ditches, which puts children and other individuals at higher risk of drowning [33]. Virtually all (95%) drowning events occurred in the daylight hours. This pattern of seasonality and time of drowning are in accordance with other studies [25,28,33,34].

A major limitation of this study is in its definition of near-drowning events. There is no standard operational definition of non-fatal drowning. In the previous 2005 BHIS survey, a non-fatal drowning event was defined as a victim who sought medical care or had at least a three-day work loss or absence from school or inability to do normal daily activities, but in the current study, it was defined just as survival from a drowning event associated with care-seeking and or at least one-day work loss or absence from school in the current study. Hence, findings on non-fatal drowning events of this study are not comparable to the BHIS study. Notwithstanding this limitation, while the absolute rates of non-fatal drowning among children less than 18 years of age in this study were different from a previous study, the drowning pattern (higher rates among this age group) was found to be similar [9].

Additionally, the study covered predominantly rural areas of Bangladesh; thus, the findings may not be generalizable to urban areas of Bangladesh. However, as the topography of rural Bangladesh is homogeneous in nature, the study findings are generalizable to other rural areas of Bangladesh.

5. Conclusions

The study suggests that the magnitude of fatal and non-fatal drowning is very high in rural communities of Bangladesh, and that drowning rates may be on the rise. Male gender, children under 5 years of age, having limited to no education, and being of lower socio-economic status were associated with increased risk of fatal and non-fatal drowning events. It is evident that drowning is a neglected public health problem in Bangladesh and that the child population is the most vulnerable. Evidence based interventions such as playpens and community crèches are effective in preventing drowning mortality in children under five years of age. It is expected that the consideration and implementation of the research findings from SoLiD will provide a wealth of knowledge in preventing child drowning. There is also a need for a national effort for drowning prevention for all ages; such an effort could incorporate other age-specific drowning prevention strategies to reduce the overall burden of drowning in rural Bangladesh.

Acknowledgments: This research was a part of the "Saving of Lives from Drowning (SoLiD) in Bangladesh" project. We thank Bloomberg Philanthropies for the kind financial support for this research activity. We gratefully acknowledge Directorate General of Health Services, Ministry of Health and Family Welfare, Government of the People's Republic of Bangladesh for their support in the study. We thank all the respondents of the study for providing their valuable time by participating in the interviews. Our special thanks to all the data collectors and supervisors for their hard work in collecting data.

Author Contributions: Aminur Rahman participated in the design, implementation, and supervision of fieldwork and analysis and wrote the paper. Olakunle Alonge and Adnan A. Hyder developed the project design, advised on project implementation, and contributed to the writing of the paper. Olakunle Alonge also contributed to the conceptualization of the paper, assisted with data analysis, and edited the manuscript for intellectual content. Al-Amin Bhuiyan and Shumona Sharmin were responsible for implementation and supervision of field activities and contributed to the writing of the paper. Priyanka Agrawal reviewed and edited the manuscript for intellectual content. Abu Talab and Qazi Sadeq-ur Rahman assisted in data management and analysis and contributed to the writing of the paper. Adnan A. Hyder is the guarantor.

Conflicts of Interest: The authors declare no conflict of interest.

References

1. Drowning Media Center. World Health Organization. Available online: http://www.who.int/mediacentre/factsheets/fs347/en/ (accessed on 2 November 2016).
2. Meddings, D.; Hyder, A.A.; Ozanne-Smith, R.A. Global Report on Drowning: Preventing a Leading Killer. Available online: http://www.who.int/violence_injury_prevention/global_report_drowning/en/ (accessed on 1 December 2016).
3. Coffman, S.P. Parent education for drowning prevention. *J. Pediatr. Health Care* **1991**, *5*, 141–146. [CrossRef]
4. MacKellar, A. Deaths from injury in childhood in Western Australia 1983–1992. *Med. J. Aust.* **1995**, *162*, 238–242. [PubMed]
5. Smith, G.S. Drowning prevention in children: The need for new strategies. *Inj. Prev.* **1995**, *1*, 216–217. [CrossRef] [PubMed]
6. Cass, D.T.; Ross, F.; Lam, L.T. Childhood drowning in New South Wales 1990–1995: A population-based study. *Med. J. Aust.* **1996**, *165*, 610–612. [PubMed]
7. Bener, A.; Al-Salman, K.M.; Pugh, R.N. Injury mortality and morbidity among children in the United Arab Emirates. *Eur. J. Epidemiol.* **1998**, *14*, 175–178. [CrossRef] [PubMed]
8. Peden, M.; Oyegbite, K.; Ozanne-smith, J.; Hyder, A.A.; Branche, C.; Rahman, A.K.M.F.; Rivara, F.; Bartolomeos, K. World Report on Child Injury Prevention. Available online: http://apps.who.int/iris/bitstream/10665/43851/1/9789241563574_eng.pdf (accessed on 5 December 2016).

9. Rahman, A.; Rahman, R.; Shafinaz, S.; Linnan, M. Bangladesh Health and Injury Survey. Available online: https://www.unicef.org/bangladesh/Bangladesh_Health_and_Injury_Survey-Report_on_Children.pdf (accessed on 5 December 2016).

10. National Institute of Population Research and Training (NIPORT); Mitra and Associates; ICF International. *Bangladesh Demographic and Health Survey 2011.* Available online: https://dhsprogram.com/pubs/pdf/fr265/fr265.pdf (accessed on 13 November 2016).

11. Kemp, A.; Sibert, J.R. Drowning and near drowning in children in the United Kingdom: Lessons of prevention. *Br. Med. J.* **1992**, *304*, 1143–1146. [CrossRef]

12. Warneke, C.L.; Cooper, S.P. Child and adolescent drowning in Harris County, Texas 1983 through 1990. *Am. J. Public Health* **1994**, *84*, 593–598. [CrossRef] [PubMed]

13. Stevenson, M.R.; Rimajova, M.; Edgecombe, D.; Vickery, K. Childhood drowning: Barriers surrounding private swimming pools. *Pediatrics* **2003**, *111*, e115–e119. [CrossRef] [PubMed]

14. Hyder, A.A.; Borse, N.N.; Blum, L.; Khan., R.; El Arifeen, S.; Baqui, A.H. Childhood drowning in low- and middle-income countries: Urgent need for intervention trials. *J. Paediatr. Child Health* **2008**, *44*, 221–227. [CrossRef] [PubMed]

15. Rahman, A.; Mashreky, S.R.; Chowdhury, S.M.; Giashuddin, M.S.; Uhaa, I.J.; Shafinaz, S. Analysis of the childhood fatal drowning situation in Bangladesh: Exploring prevention measures for low-income countries. *Inj. Prev.* **2009**, *15*, 75–79. [CrossRef] [PubMed]

16. Ma, W.J.; Nie, S.P.; Xu, H.F.; Xu, Y.J.; Song, X.L.; Guo, Q.Z.; Zhang, Y.R. An analysis of risk factors of non-fatal drowning among children in rural areas of Guangdong Province, China: A case-control study. *Int. J. Inj. Contr. Saf. Promot.* **2015**, *22*, 243–253. [CrossRef] [PubMed]

17. Hyder, A.A.; Arifeen, S.; Begum, N.; Fishman, S.; Wali, S.; Baqi, A.H. Death from drowning: Defining a new challenge for child survival in Bangladesh. *Inj. Contr. Saf. Promot.* **2003**, *10*, 205–210. [CrossRef] [PubMed]

18. Callaghan, J.A.; Hyder, A.A.; Khan, R.; Blum, L.S.; Arifeen, S.; Baqi, A.H. Child supervision practices for drowning prevention in rural Bangladesh: A pilot study of supervision tools. *J. Epidemiol. Community Health* **2010**, *64*, 645–647. [CrossRef] [PubMed]

19. Guevarra, J.P.; Franklin, R.C.; Basilio, J.A.; Orbillo, L.L.; Go, J.J. Child drowning prevention in the Philippines: The beginning of a conversation. *BMC Public Health* **2010**, *10*, 156. [CrossRef] [PubMed]

20. Laosee, O.; Khiewyoo, J.; Somrongthong, R. Drowning risk perceptions among rural guardians of Thailand: A community-based household survey. *J. Child Health Care* **2014**, *18*, 168–177. [CrossRef] [PubMed]

21. Shen, J.; Pang, S.; Schwebel, D.C. Cognitive and Behavioral Risk Factors for Unintentional Drowning among Rural Chinese Children. *Int. J. Behav. Med.* **2016**, *23*, 243–250. [CrossRef] [PubMed]

22. Rahman, F.; Bose, S.; Linnan, M.; Rahman, A.; Mashreky, S.R.; Haaland, B.; Finkelstein, E. Cost-effectiveness of an injury and drowning prevention program in Bangladesh. *Pediatrics* **2012**, *130*, e1621–e1628. [CrossRef] [PubMed]

23. World Health Organization. Global Health Estimates. Available online: http://www.who.int/healthinfo/global_burden_disease/en/ (accessed on 22 December 2016).

24. Van Beeck, E.F.; Branche, C.M.; Szpilman, D.; Modell, J.H.; Bierens, J.J.L.M. A new definition of drowning: Towards documentation and prevention of a global public health problem. *Bull. World Health Organ.* **2005**, *83*, 853–856. [PubMed]

25. Rahman, F.; Andersson, R.; Svanstrom, L. Health impact of injuries: A population-based epidemiological investigation in a local community of Bangladesh. *J. Saf. Res.* **1998**, *29*, 213–222. [CrossRef]

26. SwinSafe Preventing Child Drowning. Available online: http://swimsafe.org/swimsafe-projects/bangladesh/ (accessed on 26 January 2016).

27. Croft, J.L.; Button, C. Interacting factors associated with adult male drowning in New Zealand. *Public Lib. Sci.* **2015**, *10*, e0130545. [CrossRef] [PubMed]

28. Linnan, M.; Anh, L.V.; Cuong, P.V. Child Mortality and Injury in Asia: Survey Results and Evidence. Available online: https://www.unicef-irc.org/publications/pdf/iwp_2007_06.pdf (accessed on 26 December 2016).

29. WHO. The Injury Chart Book: A Graphical Overview of the Global Burden of Injuries. Available online: http://www.who.int/violence_injury_prevention/publications/other_injury/chartb/en/ (accessed on 31 December 2016).

30. Ahmed, M.K.; Rahman, M.; Van Ginneken, J. Epidemiology of child deaths due to drowning in Matlab, Bangladesh. *Int. J. Epidemiol.* **1999**, *28*, 306–311. [CrossRef] [PubMed]
31. Rahman, A.; Giashuddin, S.M.; Svanstrom, L.; Rahman, F. Drowning—A major but neglected child health problem in rural Bangladesh: Implications for low-income countries. *Int. J. Inj. Contr. Saf. Promot.* **2006**, *13*, 101–105. [CrossRef] [PubMed]
32. Abdullah, S.H.; Flora, M.S. Non-fatal drowning in under-five rural children of Bangladesh. *Ibrahim Med. Coll. J.* **2016**, *9*, 37–41. [CrossRef]
33. Muhuri, P.K. Estimating seasonality effects on child mortality in Matlab. *Demography* **1996**, *33*, 98–110. [CrossRef] [PubMed]
34. Baqi, A.H.; Black, R.E.; Arefeen, S.E.; Hill, K.; Mitra, S.N.; Sabir, A. Causes of childhood deaths in Bangldesh: Results of a nationwide verbal autopsy study. *Bull. World Health Organ.* **1998**, *76*, 161–171.

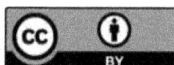

International Journal of
*Environmental Research
and Public Health*

MDPI

Article

Pattern of Road Traffic Injuries in Rural Bangladesh: Burden Estimates and Risk Factors

Md. Kamran Ul Baset [1], Aminur Rahman [1], Olakunle Alonge [2,*], Priyanka Agrawal [2], Shirin Wadhwaniya [2] and Fazlur Rahman [1]

[1]   Center for Injury Prevention and Research, Bangladesh, House # B-162, Road # 23, New DOHS, Mohakhali, Dhaka 1206, Bangladesh; kamran@ciprb.org (M.K.U.B.); aminur@ciprb.org (A.R.); fazlur@ciprb.org (F.R.)
[2]   Department of International Health, Bloomberg School of Public Health, Johns Hopkins University, Baltimore, MD 21205, USA; pagrawa6@jhu.edu (P.A.); swadhwa2@jhu.edu (S.W.)
*   Correspondence: oalonge1@jhu.edu; Tel.: +1-(443)-676-4994

Received: 5 September 2017; Accepted: 2 November 2017; Published: 7 November 2017

Abstract: Globally, road traffic injury (RTI) causes 1.3 million deaths annually. Almost 90% of all RTI deaths occur in low- and middle-income countries. RTI is one of the leading causes of death in Bangladesh; the World Health Organization estimated that it kills over 21,000 people in the country annually. This study describes the current magnitude and risk factors of RTI for different age groups in rural Bangladesh. A household census was carried out in 51 unions of seven sub-districts situated in the north and central part of Bangladesh between June and November 2013, covering 1.2 million individuals. Trained data collectors collected information on fatal and nonfatal RTI events through face-to-face interviews using a set of structured pre-tested questionnaires. The recall periods for fatal and non-fatal RTI were one year and six months, respectively. The mortality and morbidity rates due to RTI were 6.8/100,000 population/year and 889/100,000 populations/six months, respectively. RTI mortality and morbidity rates were significantly higher among males compared to females. Deaths and morbidities due to RTI were highest among those in the 25–64 years age group. A higher proportion of morbidity occurred among vehicle passengers (34%) and pedestrians (18%), and more than one-third of the RTI mortality occurred among pedestrians. Twenty percent of all nonfatal RTIs were classified as severe injuries. RTI is a major public health issue in rural Bangladesh. Immediate attention is needed to reduce preventable deaths and morbidities in rural Bangladesh.

Keywords: road traffic injuries; risk factors; epidemiology; Bangladesh

1. Introduction

There is a growing consensus in the international health community that road traffic injury (RTI) is a leading cause of death, illness, and disability throughout the world [1–3]. According to a World Health Organization (WHO) report, RTI causes 1.3 million deaths per year globally [4]. RTI death rates are more than twice as high in low- and middle-income countries (LMICs) compared to high-income countries (HICs), with almost 90% of all RTI deaths occurring in LMICs [5–9]. In LMICs, RTIs result in losses of up to 5% of the GDP compared with 3% globally [4].

Due to rapid motorization and urbanization in Bangladesh, RTIs are on the rise as in other LMICs, and RTI also represents a leading cause of injury deaths [3,10–13]. In addition to deaths, RTI is a major cause of hospital admissions at primary and secondary facilities in Bangladesh [14], and traditional data sources such as police data grossly underreport incidence of RTI events in Bangladesh. For example, police statistics showed 3160 deaths due to RTI in 2003, whereas the Bangladesh Health and Injury Survey (BHIS) reported 13,000 RTI deaths in the same year [11]. Similarly, a recent police report showed 2538 deaths due to road crashes in 2012, much lower than the 21,316 road traffic deaths estimated by the WHO [4]. More RTI deaths are recorded in the rural areas of Bangladesh compared to the urban regions [15]. According to the Road Safety Global Report (2015), Bangladesh lacks best practice legislations for all five road safety risk factors, including speeding, helmet use, drink driving, seatbelt use, and child restraint use, which make the situation even worse [4,16].

Bangladesh has had a gradual shift from infectious disease to non-communicable disease and injuries in the past couple of years [11–13,17–20]. The United Nations (UN) declared the period of 2011–2020 as a Decade of Action for Road Safety and two of the 17 Sustainable Development Goals (SDG) indicators aim to reduce global road traffic deaths and injuries by 50% by 2020, in addition to providing access to safe, affordable, accessible, and sustainable transport systems for all by 2030, which is a reflection of the growing recognition of the enormous toll exacted by RTIs [8,21,22]. However, Bangladesh has not taken any remarkable steps to address these unnecessary deaths due to the lack of reliable data on risk factors for RTI [23,24]. To design and implement comprehensive road safety strategies in Bangladesh, knowledge of the magnitude and risk factors for RTI in the country are essential. The objective of this study was to fill the current knowledge gap in RTI epidemiology and risk factors among all populations in rural Bangladesh.

2. Methods

"Saving of Lives from Drowning (SoLiD)", an implementation research study, was conducted between 2013 and 2015 in Bangladesh. In this program, a baseline census was conducted between June–November 2013 in 51 unions of seven sub-districts [25]. The seven sub-districts were Raiganj and Sherpur Sadar in the north of the country, and Matlab North, Matlab South, Daudkandi, Chandpur Sadar, and Manohardi situated in the central part of Bangladesh. The survey covered approximately 1.2 million people in 270,387 households in 993 villages of 51 unions. The survey collected information on all individuals who were residents in the survey areas.

Trained data collectors gathered required information by face-to-face interviews with the heads of households or any household member over 18 years of age who were the most knowledgeable about the household. A repeat visit was made to those households if there was no adult member present or if the respondent was physically or mentally unable to participate in the interview. If an additional second or third visit was unsuccessful, the household was excluded from the census. A set of seven pre-tested structured questionnaires was used to collect relevant information. Data was collected in two stages; the first round collected information on socioeconomic and demographic factors (sex, age, level of education, socioeconomic status), household environment, child and birth history, and health-seeking behavior to understand the household and family status. The survey also collected information on fatal and non-fatal injuries. If a specific injury mortality or morbidity was identified in first round, detailed information was collected regarding the underlying injury mechanisms in the second round. In this study, injury was defined as any external harm resulting from an assault, burn, fall, animal bite, transportation of goods and persons, cuts, poisoning, blunt objects, operating machinery, suffocation, or (near) drowning resulting in the loss of one or more days of normal daily activities, work, or school, and its methodology is described elsewhere [17]. This paper only looked at fatal and non-fatal RTI outcomes. The recall periods for fatal and non-fatal RTIs were one year and six months, respectively.

To ensure the data quality, trained supervisors observed 10% of the conducted interviews and checked 10% of the collected data. They also re-interviewed 2% of the visited households. Field-level research officers also re-checked all data for inconsistencies. If any discrepancy was found, the household was revisited to collect correct information.

A data entry program using SQL Server 2008 was developed and collected data were entered, and then transferred to SPSS version 21 for analysis. All related information of fatal and non-fatal RTIs were retrieved from the primary database for analysis and were de-identified. To analyze the characteristics of RTIs, standard descriptive statistics were used. Description of population by fatal and non-fatal RTIs, sex, age, level of education, socioeconomic status (SES), and sub-district, as well as the place, time, and prior activities of fatal and non-fatal RTIs was provided with proportion.

Nonfatal injury events were classified into low, medium, and highly severe injuries based on an index that summarizes indicators such as the number of days an individual required assistance, the number of days lost at work or school, post injury immobility, anatomic and physiologic profile of an injury, post injury hospitalization, surgical treatment, and post injury disability for all events [17]. Fatal RTI rates were calculated per 100,000 population per year and non-fatal RTI rates per 100,000 population per six months. These rates were further analyzed by age, sex, SES, education, and sub-district levels.

Odds of fatal and nonfatal RTI outcomes given independent variables such as age, sex, SES, education, and occupation were assessed using logistic regressions. Results from both bivariate and multivariate logistic regressions are presented. Age was treated as a categorical variable (comprising eight groups: <5 (reference group), 5–9, 10–14, 15–17, 18–24, 25–64, 65+ years). Sex was considered as a binary predictor (reference group was female). Educational (A level and above as a reference group), occupation (agriculture as a reference group), and SES (from lowest to highest) were categorical variables.

Ethical Statement

Ethical clearance was obtained from the Institutional Review Boards of the Johns Hopkins Bloomberg School of Public Health (approval code: 00004746), International Centre for Diarrheal Disease Research, Bangladesh and the Center for Injury Prevention Research, Bangladesh. For inclusion in the study, informed consent was given by all respondent before they participated.

3. Results

3.1. Sociodemographic Characteristics of Survey Population

Around 1.2 million people from seven selected sub-districts were covered in the census, and the proportion of the population in each sub-district varied depending upon the number of unions covered for the census. In the census, the proportion of males (48.5%) and females (51.5%) were almost equal. Among the total sample, 39.1% were children (<18 years). A total of 6303 deaths (preceding year) and 119,669 non-fatal injury events (preceding six months) were identified during the census (Table 1). A total of 80 fatal RTIs (8.7% of injury death) and 10,398 non-fatal RTIs (17.8% of injury morbidity) were recorded (Table 2). Of the total, 7.4% of RTIs cases had multiple events.

Table 1. Sociodemographic characteristics of fatal and non-fatal road traffic injury (RTI) outcomes.

Characteristics	Total Population (*n* = 1,169,594)		Characteristics	Total Population (*n* = 1,169,594)	
	n	(%)		*n*	(%)
Population by Upazila			Education		
Matlab North	265,897	(22.7)	No education	295,314	(25.3)
Matlab South	209,772	(17.9)	Primary	407,923	(34.9)
Chadpur Sadar	128,356	(11.0)	Secondary	289,658	(24.8)
Raiganj	104,357	(8.9)	A levels and above	63,873	(5.5)
Sherpur	228,519	(19.5)	Not applicable (Under 5 years)	112,664	(9.6)
Manohardi	204,319	(17.5)	SES quintiles		
Daud Kandi	28,373	(2.4)	Lowest	211,601	(18.1)
			Low	218,695	(18.7)
Sex			Middle	238,371	(20.4)
Male	567,674	(48.5)	High	247,716	(21.2)
Female	601,919	(51.5)	Highest	253,210	(21.7)
Age			Occupation		
<5 years	112,664	(9.6)	Agriculture	104,956	(9.0)
5–9 years	139,728	(12.0)	Business	61,661	(5.3)
10–14 years	142,121	(12.2)	Skilled labor (Professional)	89,151	(7.7)
15–17 years	62,098	(5.3)	Unskilled/domestic (Unskilled)	24,520	(2.1)
18–24 years	133,534	(11.4)	Rickshaw/bus (Transport worker)	17,037	(1.5)
25–64 years	508,059	(43.4)	Student	312,537	(26.7)
65+ years	71,389	(6.1)	Retired/unemployed/housewife	408,583	(34.9)
			Other	150,402	(12.4)

Table 2. Fatal and non-fatal RTI rates (per 100,000) by sub-districts, sex, age, level of education, SES index, and occupation.

Characteristics	Fatal Road Traffic Injuries (n = 80)		Non-Fatal Road Traffic (n = 10,398 Events)	
	n = 80	Rate/100,000/Year (95% CI)	n = 10,398	Rate/100,000/Six Months (95% CI)
All	80	6.8	10,398	889
Upazila				
Matlab North	15	5.6 (3.4–9.3)	2405	904.5 (869.2–941.2)
Matlab South	9	4.3 (2.3–8.2)	1808	861.9 (823.2–902.4)
Chadpur Sadar	6	4.7 (2.1–10.2)	959	747.1 (701.5–795.7)
Raiganj	11	10.5 (5.9–18.9)	1595	1528.4 (1456.0–1605.0)
Sherpur	16	7.0 (4.3–11.4)	1401	613.1 (581.9–645.9)
Manohardi	21	10.3 (6.7–15.7)	2037	996.9 (954.8–1041.0)
Daudkandi	2	7.1 (1.9–25.7)	193	680.0 (591.0–782.8)
Sex				
Male	52	9.2 (6.9–12.01)	8705	1551.4 (1520.0–1584.0)
Female	28	4.7 (3.2–6.7)	1693	264.3 (251.7–277.6)
Age				
<5 years	5	4.4 (1.9–10.4)	355	315.1 (284.0–349.6)
5–9 years	8	5.7 (2.9–11.3)	1007	720.7 (677.7–766.4)
10–14 years	5	3.5 (1.5–8.2)	1048	737.4 (94.2–783.2)
15–17 years	5	8.1 (3.4–18.9)	663	1067.7 (989.8–1152.0)
18–24 years	9	6.7 (3.5–12.8)	1347	1008.7 (956.5–1064.0)
25–64 years	38	7.5 (5.45–10.3)	5510	1084.5 (1056.0–1113.0)
65+ years	10	14.0 (7.6–25.8)	468	655.6 (599.0–717.5)
Education				
No education	26	8.8 (6.0–12.9)	2708	916.9 (883.2–952.0)
Primary	21	5.2 (3.4–7.9)	3627	889.1 (860.8–918.4)
Secondary	23	7.9 (5.3–11.9)	2891	998.1 (962.5–1035)
Higher secondary and above	5	7.8(3.3–18.3)	817	1279.1 (1195.0–1369.0)
Not applicable (Under 5 years)	5	4.4 (1.9–10.4)	355	315.1 (284.0–349.6)
SES quintiles				
Lowest	18	8.5 (5.4–13.5)	1847	872.9 (834.1–913.4)
Low	13	5.9(3.5–10.2)	2006	917.3 (878.2–942.1)
Middle	14	5.9 (3.5–9.9)	1937	812.6 (777.3–849.4)
High	22	8.9 (5.9–13.5)	2131	863.8 (828.0–901.0)
Highest	13	5.1 (3.0–8.8)	2477	998.3 (940.7–1017.0)
Occupation				
Agriculture	11	10.4 (5.8–18.6)	1301	1231.1 (1166.0–1299.0)
Business	6	9.7 (4.4–21.1)	1282	2066.9 (1958.0–2182.0)
Skilled labor (Professional)	11	12.2 (6.8–21.8)	1533	1698.6 (1616.0–1785.0)
Unskilled/domestic (Unskilled)	3	12.1 (4.1–35.5)	332	1335.3 (1200.0–1486.0)
Rickshaw/bus (Transport worker)	8	46.1 (23.3–90.9)	1239	7133.0 (6760.0–7525.0)
Student	15	4.8 (2.9–7.9)	2439	774.4 (744.4–805.6)
Retired/unemployed/housewife	19	4.6 (3.0–7.2)	1575	383.1 (364.7–402.4)
Other	1	17.2 (3.0–97.1)	45	771.9 (577.4–1031.0)
Not applicable	6	4.1 (1.9–9.0)	634	435.9 (403.4–471.1)

3.2. RTI Mortality and Morbidity

RTI deaths comprised about 1.3% of the deaths that occurred due to any cause in the surveyed population over a recall period of one year. The mortality rate due to RTI was 6.8 (95% CI 55–85) per 100,000 populations per year. The mortality rate was the highest in Raiganj (10.5 per 100,000; 95% CI 5.9–18.9) followed closely by Manohardi (10.3 per 100,000; 95% CI 6.7–15.7).

Across gender profiles, RTI deaths were significantly more in males than females, the mortality rates being 9.2 deaths (95% CI 6.9–12.01) per 100,000 in males compared to 4.7 deaths (95% CI 3.2–6.7) per 100,000 in females. The count of deaths due to RTI was highest in the 25–64 years age group; the unadjusted mortality rate was, however, highest among the elderly age group (14 deaths per 100,000; 95% CI 7.1–26.7) (Table 2). Individuals with no education had the most number of RTI deaths (8.8 per 100,000; 95% CI 6.0–12.9). People with secondary and higher secondary level or higher education had similar mortality rates (Table 2).

The morbidity rate due to RTI was 889 injuries (95% CI 866–900) per 100,000 population per six months. The RTI morbidity rate was highest in Raiganj (1528.4 injuries per 100,000; 95% CI 1456–1605), followed by Manohardi (996.9 injuries per 100,000; 95% CI 954.8–1041 (Table 2). Males suffered significantly higher numbers of injuries than females across all ages, with the morbidity rate being 1551.4 injuries (95% CI 1520–1584) per 100,000 for males versus 264.3 injuries (95% CI 251.7–277.6) per 100,000 for females (Table 2). Adults aged 25 to 64 years sustained the most number of injuries, and also had the highest morbidity rate, 1084.5 injuries (95% CI 1056–1113) per 100,000 population. Adolescents and young adults followed closely, with morbidity rates of 1067.7 injuries (95% CI 989.8–1152) per 100,000 and 1084.5 injuries (1056–1113) per 100,000 population, respectively (Table 2). A higher rate of fatal RTI (8.8/100,000; 95% CI 6.0–12.9) was observed among those who were not educated compared to those with some formal education; however, the differences were not statistically significant (Table 2). In the case of non-fatal RTI events, individuals with higher secondary level and advanced education had significantly higher rates (1279.1/100,000; 95% CI 1195.0–1369.0) of RTI than individuals with lower levels or no education.

With the decrease of the SES index, the rates of fatal RTIs increased with an exception in the high SES quintile, where the rate was found to be the highest (8.9/100,000; 95% CI 5.9–13.5). However, rates of non–fatal RTIs where highest (998.3/100,000; 95% CI 940.7–1017.0) in the highest SES quintile (Table 2).

Transport workers had the highest rates for both RTI mortality (46.1/100,000; 95% CI 23.3–90.9) and morbidity (7133.0; 95% CI 6760.0–7525.0) among all occupations (Table 2). When considering the mode of transport, most victims of RTI morbidity were passengers (34%) and pedestrians (18%) (Figure 1). Most RTI mortality, however, occurred among pedestrians (35%). Auto-rickshaw, pickup van, jeep, microbus, bus, bicycle, and motorcycle were the main modes of transportation that an individual was using prior to death resulting from RTI (Figure 2).

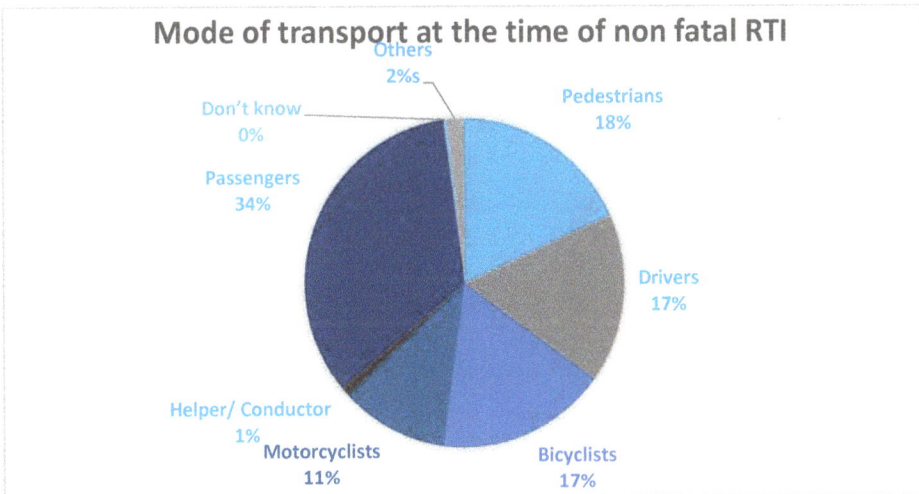

Figure 1. Mode of transport at the time of non-fatal RTI.

Mode of transport at the time of fatal RTI

Pedestrian, 35.0%

Other, 7.5%

Steamer/Launch, 6.3%

Bus/Mini bus, 8.8%

Truck, 3.8%

Informal vehicle, 3.8%

Auto – rickshawTempo/pick – up/Jeep/Microbus, 16.3%

Motorcycle, 7.5%

Rickshaw/Van, 2.5%

Bicycle, 8.8%

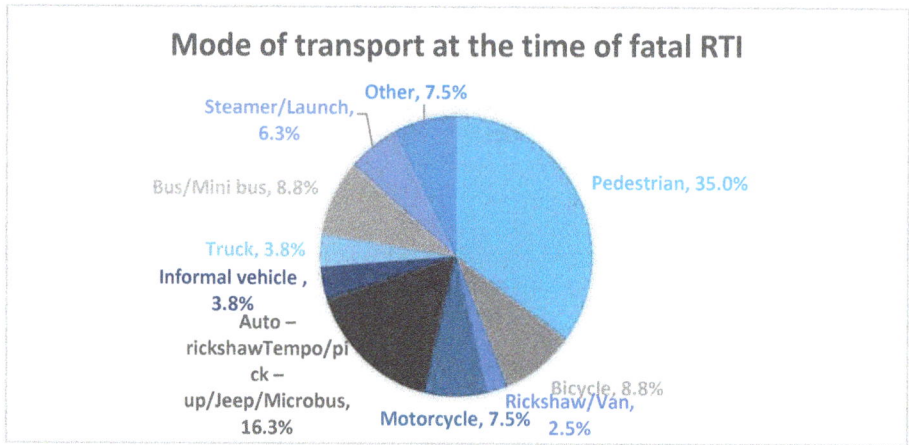

Figure 2. Mode of transport at the time of fatal RTI.

Around 40.0% of road traffic injuries occurred while an individual was on his way to work, and 21.5% occurred among individuals who were wandering on the streets. One-fifth of the victims were engaged in driving (Figure 3).

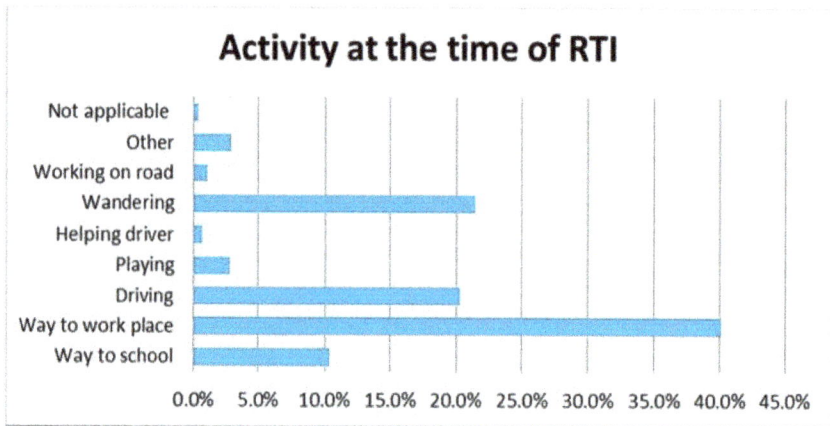

Activity at the time of RTI

Not applicable
Other
Working on road
Wandering
Helping driver
Playing
Driving
Way to work place
Way to school

0.0% 5.0% 10.0% 15.0% 20.0% 25.0% 30.0% 35.0% 40.0% 45.0%

Figure 3. Activity at the time of RTI (both mortality and morbidity).

The RTI injury severity index showed that 50% of RTI cases had low severity. Almost 20% of cases had been severely injured in a road traffic crash. The highest proportion of high injury severity was found among passengers (37.7%), followed by pedestrians (22.4%) (Figure 4).

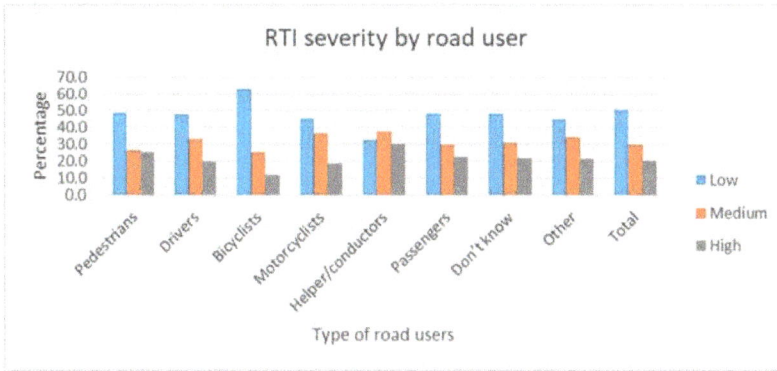

Figure 4. Injury severity index related to road user in RTI morbidity.

The survey findings revealed that 81.4% of motorcyclist RTI victims did not use safety devices (Table 3).

Table 3. Use of safety device at the time of RTI among motorcyclists.

Motorcycle user	Use of Safety Device at the Time of RTI among Motorcyclists		
	Used	Not Used	Did Not Know
	n (%)	*n* (%)	*n* (%)
Morbidity	222 (10.6)	1832 (87.9)	31 (1.5)
Mortality	1 (25.0)	3 (75.0)	0 (0.0)
Total	223 (17.8)	1835 (81.4)	31 (0.7)

Most of RTIs happened earlier in the day, between 9:00 a.m. and 12 noon (Figure 5). Most of the respondents (95.4%) mentioned that the injured person was not on drugs. It was also noted that most collisions happened between auto-rickshaws or other informal vehicles (modified vehicles, which have no legal permission to be on the road). Most (46.5%) of the respondents perceived that the road condition was not good.

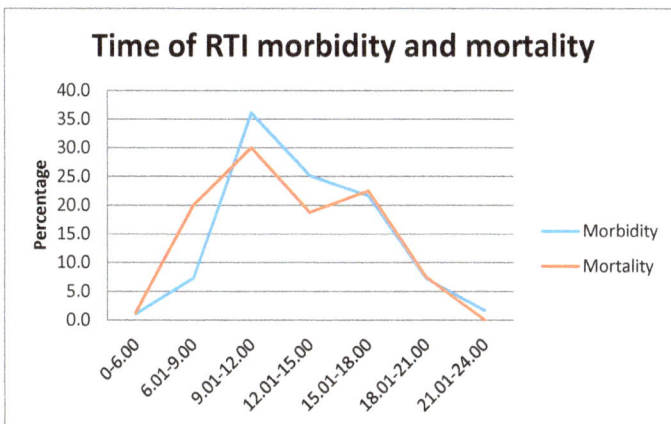

Figure 5. Time of RTI morbidity and mortality.

21

Multiple logistic regression analysis revealed that males were 4.6 times more at risk of non-fatal RTI (95% CI 4.3–4.9; p = 0.000) when compared with females. The risk of a non-fatal road traffic crash increased significantly with increasing age. Individuals aged 15 to 24 years were at the highest risk. Transport workers, such as those driving rickshaws and buses, were 6 times likelier to be in a non-fatal RTI (95% CI 5.5–6.5; p = 0.000) than agricultural workers. Education level was not seen to be associated with non-fatal RTI risk. Increasing socioeconomic status was significantly associated with increasing risk of non-fatal RTI (Table 4).

Table 4. Association between sociodemographic factors and fatal and non-fatal RTI.

Characteristics	Fatal RTI				Non-Fatal RTI			
	OR (95% CI) Unadjusted	p Value	OR (95% CI) Adjusted	p Value	OR (95% CI) Unadjusted	p Value	OR (95% CI) Adjusted	p Value
Sex								
Male	2.0 (1.2–3.1)	0.004	1.3 (0.7–2.6)	0.436	5.9 (5.6–6.2)	0.000	4.6 (4.3–4.9)	0.000
Female	1		1					
Age Groups								
<5 years	1		1					
5–9 years	1.3 (0.4–3.9)	0.655	0.5 (0.1–1.5)	0.217	2.3 (2.0–2.6)	0.000	2.9 (2.4–3.5)	0.000
10–14 years	0.8 (0.2–2.7)	0.713	0.7 (0.2–2.6)	0.207	2.3(2.1–2.6)	0.000	3.0 (2.4–3.6)	0.000
15–17 years	1.8 (0.5–6.3)	0.346	0.5 (0.1–2.0)	0.625	3.4 (3.0–3.9)	0.000	3.8 (3.1–4.6)	0.000
18–24 years	1.5 (0.5–4.5)	0.454	0.5 (0.1–1.8)	0.343	3.2 (2.9–3.6)	0.000	3.7 (3.1–4.5)	0.000
25–64 years	1.7 (0.7–4.3)	0.273	1.3 (0.3–4.8)	0.297	3.4 (3.1–3.8)	0.000	3.7 (3.0–4.5)	0.000
65+ years	3.2 (1.1–9.2)	0.036	0.5 (0.1–1.5)	0.742	2.2 (1.9–2.5)	0.000	2.8 (2.3–3.5)	0.000
Level of education								
Not applicable	0.6 (0.2–2.0)	0.370	0.7 (0.4–1.4)	0.573	0.2 (0.2–0.3)	0.000		
No education	1.1 (0.4–2.9)	0.810	1.3 (0.7–2.5)	0.312	0.7 (0.7–0.8)	0.000	0.9 (0.8–1.0)	0.110
Primary	0.7 (0.2–1.7)	0.400	1.1 (0.3–4.1)	0.475	0.7 (0.6–0.7)	0.000	0.9 (0.9–1.0)	0.118
Secondary	1.0 (0.4–2.7)	0.977	1.0 (0.1–8.2)	0.900	0.8 (0.7–0.8)	0.000	1.0 (0.9–1.1)	0.794
Higher secondary and above	1		1		1		1	
Occupation								
Agriculture	1		1					
Business	0.9 (0.3–2.5)	0.884	1.4 (0.4–2.8)	0.004	1.7 (1.6–1.8)	0.000	1.6 (1.5–1.7)	0.000
Skilled labourer	1.2 (0.5–2.7)	0.702	1.2 (0.5–3.1)	0.969	1.4 (1.3–1.5)	0.000	1.4 (1.3–1.5)	0.000
Unskilled/domestic worker	1.2 (0.3–4.2)	0.812	1.3 (0.4–4.7)	0.636	1.1 (1.0–1.2)	0.184	1.2 (1.1–1.4)	0.004
Transport worker (Rickshaw/bus)	4.5 (1.8–11.1)	0.001	5.1 (2.0–13.0)	0.000	6.2 (5.7–6.7)	0.000	6.0 (5.5–6.5)	0.000
Student	0.5(0.2–1.0)	0.049	0.8 (0.1–1.7)	0.001	0.6(0.6–0.7)	0.000	1.1 (1.0–1.2)	0.067
Retired/unemployed/housewife	0.4 (0.2–0.9)	0.032	0.5 (0.2–1.4)	0.277	0.3 (0.3–0.3)	0.000	1.0 (0.9–1.1)	0.397
Not applicable (children)	0.4 (0.1–1.1)	0.068	1.2 (0.0–2.5)	0.201	0.4 (0.3–0.4)	0.000	1.3 (1.1–1.6)	0.000
Not applicable (other)	1.6 (0.2–12.4	0.651	1.2 (0.1–9.9)	0.228	0.6 (0.5–0.8)	0.002	1.2 (0.9–1.7)	0.164
SES index								
Lowest	1							
Low	0.7 (0.3–1.4)	0.325	0.8 (0.4–1.6)	0.681	1.1 (1.0–1.1)	0.132	1.1 (1.0–1.1)	0.067
Middle	0.7 (0.3–1.4)	0.299	0.7 (0.3–1.4)	0.493	0.9 (0.9–1.0)	0.026	0.9 (0.9–1.0)	0.125
High	1.0 (0.6–1.9)	0.892	1.0 (0.5–2.0)	0.289	1.0 (0.9–1.0)	0.654	1.0 (0.9–1.1)	0.855
Highest	0.6 (0.3–1.2)	0.165	0.7 (0.3–1.5)	0.986	1.1 (1.1–1.2)	0.000	1.2 (1.1–1.3)	0.000

With fatal RTI cases, gender and age were not significantly associated with an increased risk of death due to an RTI. As with non-fatal RTI events, transport workers were 4.5 times more (95% CI 1.8–11.1) at risk than agricultural workers to die in a road traffic accident (Table 4).

4. Discussion

The incidence of RTI fatalities was found to be 6.8 deaths (95% CI 55–85) per 100,000 population and non-fatal RTIs were calculated as 889.0 injuries (95% CI 866–900) per 100,000 population. Although RTIs occur in all age groups, the highest rate of fatality (14.0 per 100,000 population) was observed among the older age group (65+ years) followed by 15–17 years (8.1 per 100,000 population), and the highest rate of morbidity was found in the group aged in 24–64 years (1084.4 per 100,000 population). These findings were consistent with other studies from the developing world such as India, Pakistan, Nepal, Vietnam, and Ghana, where RTI was found to be the leading killer and the productive age group was found to be the most likely victim [26–32]. Other studies also showed that the most active and productive age group, 15–35 years, was the most likely victim of RTI deaths [1,28,33–35]. This enhances a serious economic loss to the country, thereby affecting the growth of the county. The reasons behind this trend may be that children have less mobility and are also supervised by adults during road use, but adults have more mobility and exposure to road traffic in order to attend work and studies [36].

Male preponderance in fatal and non-fatal RTIs is concurrent with other studies from Bangladesh and the surrounding countries [7,14,37–39]. This is probably because men in Bangladesh have more exposure and movement on the road due to their involvement in work, business, jobs, or studies, whereas females are often restricted to their homes and are responsible for handling household chores [40].

The study findings noticed that no education and lower socioeconomic conditions put individuals at higher risk for road traffic injury deaths. Other studies conducted in LMICs and HICs found similar patterns [11,13,14,36,39–43]. Moreover, the Global Status Report of Road Traffic Injury also projected that poor socioeconomic condition will have a significant role in RTIs and people from a lower socioeconomic status are more likely to be affected [4]. SES is an important predictor for health conditions, especially in RTI situations. RTI is an acute health problem; however, immediate proper health care is not available for poor people in LMICs [4,9,11,15].

In this study, mortality and morbidity were highest among transport workers, such as rickshaw pullers. It has been reported in different studies that more RTIs were seen among students and laborers [14,44–46]. The open design of a rickshaw could be one reason why such rickshaw pullers are at higher risk [47]. It is interesting to note that passengers were more involved in non-fatal RTIs, whereas pedestrians were involved in deadly RTIs. Similar findings have been highlighted in many other studies in LMICs [10,15]. Pedestrians appear to be at greater risk of death and injury due to RTI. This could be clarified by the fact that people mostly travel on foot in rural areas of Bangladesh and these areas are not equipped with properly designed roads. This puts pedestrians at a higher risk of being knocked down by motor vehicles [48]. Most of the studies in LMICs showed the same picture of RTIs, in that pedestrian are predominantly affected by road traffic crashes owing to the mixture of slow and fast vehicles in addition to pedestrians on the same roads [49–52]. It was also noted that most of the collisions happened between auto-rickshaws or other informal three-wheelers, which are the main vehicles used on rural roads [15,35,48].

In the present study, the highest number of crashes happened between morning and noon (9 a.m. to 12 p.m.). This pattern is similar to other studies from Bangladesh and the surrounding regions, such as India, where the highest incidence of RTIs occurred in the same time frame [11,16]. These are the peak hours for traffic on the roads, as children go to school and adults head to their work places [11,15,52]. Motorcyclists who did not use helmets were the most severely injured. Similar findings for the lack of helmet use was also found in other studies [12,17,52].

The strength of this study is that data was collected from a large sample size covering all individuals in the survey area. The information was collected through two-stage verbal interviews by trained data collectors and all data was cross-checked. However, data was collected mostly from rural areas of Bangladesh; therefore, the findings may not be generalizable to urban areas of Bangladesh and these sample households were not nationally representative [4]. However, the topography, road networks, and road structures of rural Bangladesh are similar in nature, thus the study outcomes are generalizable to other areas of rural Bangladesh [15].

Additionally, the study did not collect data on other risk factors such as exposure time, kilometers driven, and knowledge of safety practices. Furthermore, not all respondents were victims or eye witnesses, which gives some limitation to data accuracy.

Other established common risk factors such as lack of awareness, lack of engineering modification, and travelling on overcrowded or poorly maintained vehicles could not be captured in the context of this study.

5. Conclusions

The magnitude of fatal and non-fatal RTIs is remarkably high in rural communities of Bangladesh, and the working age group and male population are more at risk. Being a pedestrian or a student were also identified as risk factors for both fatal and non-fatal RTIs. Lower socioeconomic condition and no education were the important risk factors for fatal and non-fatal RTIs.

There is obviously a need for targeted and directed intervention approaches to reduce road traffic injuries. Some examples of interventions include road safety education programs for road users, safe child pedestrian programs through school education, community awareness programs, first responder training at the community level, the implementation of safety measures for non-motorized vehicles, and engineering modifications for speed calming. Such approaches should be directed towards vulnerable road users [15,19,46,51]. Immediate attention should be made to strengthen the intervention measures in an integrated manner to prevent these unexpected events.

Acknowledgments: We would like to acknowledge Bloomberg Philanthropies for their kind support and for providing the funding to implement the SoLiD study in Bangladesh. We would like to thank our partners, Johns Hopkins University Bloomberg School of Public Health and International Center for Diarrheal Disease Research, Bangladesh for their invaluable expertise and support in helping us implement the project. We would also thank all the respondents of the study for providing their valuable time by participating in the interviews as well as the SoLiD field team for their hard work in collecting data.

Author Contributions: Md. Kamran Ul Baset and Olakunle Alonge conceived the paper, Kamran contributed to the supervision of field work, data analysis, wrote the initial drafts of the manuscript, and reviewed the final draft for intellectual content. Aminur Rahman, Olakunle Alonge, Shirin Wadhwaniya, Fazlur Rahman, and Priyanka Agrawal contributed to the review of data analysis and editing the final draft of the manuscript for intellectual content. All co-authors provided editing support in finalizing the manuscript.

Conflicts of Interest: The authors declare no conflict of interest.

Abbreviations

RTI	road traffic incident
LMIC	low- and middle-income country
HIC	high-income country
CIPRB	Center for Injury Prevention and Research, Bangladesh (CIRPB)
Icddr,b	International Center for Diarrheal Disease Research, Bangladesh (icddr,b)
CI	Confidence Interval

References

1. Peden, M.; Scurfield, R.; Sleet, D.; Mohan, D.; Hyder, A.; Jarawan, E.; Mathers, C. *World Report on Road Traffic Injury Prevention*; World Health Organization: Geneva, Switzerland, 2014; Available online: http://cdrwww.who.int/entity/violence_injury_prevention/publications/road_traffic/world_report/intro.pdf (accessed on 21 June 2016).
2. Ma, W.J.; Nie, S.P.; Xu, H.F.; Xu, Y.J.; Zhang, Y.R. Socioeconomic status and the occurrence of non-fatal child pedestrian injury: Results from a cross-sectional survey. *Saf. Sci.* **2010**, *48*, 823–828. [CrossRef]
3. Staton, C.; Vissoci, J.; Gong, E.; Toomey, N.; Wafula, R.; Abdelgadir, J.; Zhou, Y.; Liu, C.; Pei, F.; Zick, B.Z.; et al. Road traffic injury prevention initiatives: A systematic review and metasummary of effectiveness in low and middle income countries. *PLoS ONE* **2016**, *11*, e0144971.
4. World Health Organization. *Global Status Reports on Road Safety 2015*; World Health Organization: Geneva, Switzerland, 2015; Available online: http://www.who.int/violence_injury_prevention/road_safety_status/2015/en (accessed on 21 June 2016).
5. Peden, M. Global collaboration on road traffic injury prevention. *Int. J. Inj. Control Saf. Promot.* **2005**, *12*, 85–91. [CrossRef] [PubMed]
6. Hyder, A.A.; Peden, M. Inequality and road-traffic injuries: Call for action. *Lancet* **2003**, *362*, 2034–2035. [CrossRef]
7. Hyder, A.A.; Amach, O.H.; Garg, N.; Labinjo, M.T. Estimating the burden of road traffic injuries among children and adolescents in urban South Asia. *Health Policy* **2006**, *77*, 129–139. [CrossRef] [PubMed]
8. World Health Organization. Ensuring the Decade is Action: UN Decade of Action for Road Safety 2011–2020. Available online: http://www.makeroadssafe.org/publications/Documents/decade_is_action_booklet.pdf (accessed on 7 September 2011).

9. Naci, H.; Chisholm, D.; Baker, T.D. Distribution of road traffic deaths by road user group: A global comparison. *Inj. Prev.* **2009**, *15*, 55–59. [CrossRef] [PubMed]
10. Uz Zaman, A.H.; Alam, K.M.T.; Islam, M.J. Urbanization in Bangladesh: Present Status and Policy Implication. *ASA Univ. Rev.* **2010**, *4*. Available online: https://pdfs.semanticscholar.org/4595/65a90508347585e3030c20a67153078af7cb.pdf (accessed on 21 June 2016).
11. Rahman, A.; Rahman, F.; Shafinaz, S.; Linnan, M. *Bangladesh Health and Injury Survey: Report on Children*; DGHS; ICMH; Unicef; TASC: Dhaka, Bangladesh, 2005.
12. Mashreky, S.R.; Rahman, A.; Chowdhury, S.M.; Giashuddin, S.; SvanstrÖm, L.; Linnan, M.; Shafinaz, S.; Uhaa, I.J.; Rahman, F. Epidemiology of childhood burn: Yield of largest community based injury survey in Bangladesh. *Burns* **2008**, *34*, 856–862. [CrossRef] [PubMed]
13. Dalal, K.; Rahman, A. Out-of-pocket payments for unintentional injuries: A study in rural Bangladesh. *Int. J. Inj. Control Saf. Promot.* **2009**, *16*, 41–47. [CrossRef] [PubMed]
14. Mashreky, S.R.; Rahman, A.; Khan, T.F.; Faruque, M.; Svanström, L.; Rahman, F. Hospital burden of road traffic injury: Major concern in primary and secondary level hospitals in Bangladesh. *Public Health* **2010**, *124*, 185–189. [CrossRef] [PubMed]
15. Baset, M. Road Traffic Injury Prevention in Children in Rural Bangladesh (Doctoral Dissertation, University of the West of England). 2013. Available online: http://eprints.uwe.ac.uk/22643 (accessed on 15 April 2016).
16. Alonge, O.; Agrawal, P.; Talab, A.; Rahman, Q.S.; Rahman, A.F.; El Arifeen, S.; Hyder, A.A. Fatal and non-fatal injury outcomes: Results from a purposively sampled census of seven rural subdistricts in Bangladesh. *Lancet Glob. Health* **2017**, *5*, e818–e827. [CrossRef]
17. Aeron-Thomas, A.; Jacobs, G.D.; Sexton, B.; Gururaj, G.; Rahman, F. *The Involvement and Impact of Road Crashes on the Poor: Bangladesh and India Case Studies*; Report Number: PPR 10; TRL Limited: London, UK, 2010. Available online: https://assets.publishing.service.gov.uk/media/57a08cbced915d622c001533/R7780.pdf (accessed on 21 June 2016).
18. Rahman, F.; Andersson, R.; Svanström, L. Medical help seeking behaviour of injury patients in a community in Bangladesh. *Public Health* **1998**, *112*, 31–35. [CrossRef]
19. Chowdhury, S.M.; Rahman, A.; Mashreky, S.R.; Giashuddin, S.; SvanstrÖm, L.; Hortel, L.G.; Rahman, F. The Horizon of Unintentional Injuries among Children in Low-Income Setting: An Overview from Bangladesh Health and Injury Survey. *J. Environ. Public Health* **2009**, 1–6. Available online: http://downloads.hindawi.com/journals/jeph/2009/435403.pdf (accessed on 21 June 2016). [CrossRef] [PubMed]
20. Ahsan, K.Z.; Alam, N.; Streatfield, K.P. Epidemiological transition in rural Bangladesh, 1986–2006. *Glob. Health Action* **2009**, *2*, 1904. [CrossRef] [PubMed]
21. WHO. *Global Status Report on Road Safety 2013: Supporting a Decade of Action*; World Health Organization: Geneva, Switzerland, 2013. Available online: https://books.google.com/books?hl=en&lr=&id=rrMXDAAAQBAJ&oi=fnd&pg=PP1&dq=22.%09WHO.+Global+Status+Report+on+Road+Safety+2013:+Supporting+a+Decade+of+Action.+Luxembourg:+World+Health+Organisation.+2013&ots=MELS7G7bal&sig=Z06hioYegDuwV0XyCyAhsMDB-MQ (accessed on 7 September 2016).
22. Resolution Adopted by the General Assembly on 15 April 2016 (Without Reference to a Main Committee (A/70/L.44 and Add.1)) 70/260. Improving Global Road Safety, Seventieth Session Agenda Item 13, UN General Assemble. 2016. Available online: http://www.who.int/violence_injury_prevention/media/news/2016/15_04/en (accessed on 6 September 2016).
23. Krug, E. Decade of action for road safety 2011–2020. *Injury* **2012**, *43*, 6–7. [CrossRef] [PubMed]
24. Romão, F.; Nizamo, H.; Mapasse, D.; Rafico, M.M.; José, J.; Mataruca, S.; Efron, M.L.; Omondi, L.O.; Leifert, T.; Bicho, J.M.L.M. Road traffic injuries in Mozambique. *Inj. Control Saf. Promot.* **2003**, *10*, 63–67. [PubMed]
25. He, S.; Alonge, O.; Agrawal, P.; Sharmin, S.; Islam, I.; Mashreky, S.R.; Arifeen, S.E. Epidemiology of burns in rural Bangladesh: An update. *Int. J. Environ. Res. Public Health* **2017**, *14*, 381. [CrossRef] [PubMed]
26. Rodríguez, D.Y.; Fernández, F.J.; Velásquez, H.A. Road traffic injuries in Colombia. *Inj. Control Saf. Promot.* **2003**, *10*, 29–35. [PubMed]
27. Odero, W.; Khayesi, M.; Heda, P.M. Road traffic injuries in Kenya: Magnitude, causes and status of intervention. *Inj. Control Saf. Promot.* **2003**, *10*, 53–61. [CrossRef] [PubMed]
28. St. Bernard, G.; Matthews, W. A contemporary analysis of road traffic crashes, fatalities and injuries in Trinidad and Tobago. *Inj. Control Saf. Promot.* **2003**, *10*, 21–27. [CrossRef] [PubMed]

29. Poudel-Tandukar, K.; Nakahara, S.; Ichikawa, M.; Poudel, K.C.; Joshi, A.B.; Wakai, S. Unintentional injuries among school adolescents in Kathmandu, Nepal: A descriptive study. *Public Health* **2006**, *120*, 641–649. [CrossRef] [PubMed]

30. Dandona, R.; Kumar, G.; Ameer, M.; Ahmed, G.; Dandona, L. Incidence and burden of road traffic injuries in urban India. *Inj. Prev.* **2008**, *14*, 354–359. [CrossRef] [PubMed]

31. Labinjo, M.; Juillard, C.; Kobusingye, O.C.; Hyder, A.A. The burden of road traffic injuries in Nigeria: Results of a population-based survey. *Inj. Prev.* **2009**, *15*, 157–162. [CrossRef] [PubMed]

32. Kiran, E.; Saralaya, K.; Vijaya, K. Prospective study on road traffic accidents. *J. Punjab Acad. Forensic Med. Toxicol.* **2004**, *4*, 12–16.

33. Verma, P.K.; Tiwari, K.N. Epidemiology of Road Traffic Injuries in Delhi: Result of a Survey. *Reg. Health Forum* **2004**, *8*, 6–14.

34. Rahman, A. *Epidemiology of Road Traffic Injury in Bangladesh. 22–24th August*; Accident Research Centre: Melbourne, Victoria, Australia, 2006.

35. Jha, N.; Srinivasa, D.K.; Roy, G.; Jagdish, S.; Minocha, R.K. Epidemiological study of road traffic accident cases: A study from South India. *Indian J. Community Med.* **2004**, *29*, 20–24.

36. Sharma, B.R. Road traffic injuries: A major global public health crisis. *Public Health* **2008**, *122*, 1399–1406. [CrossRef] [PubMed]

37. Patil, S.S.; Kakade, R.V.; Durgawale, P.M.; Kakade, S.V. Pattern of road traffic injuries: A study from western Maharashtra. *Indian J. Community Med.* **2008**, *33*, 56–57. [CrossRef] [PubMed]

38. Dandona, R.; Kumar, G.A.; Raj, T.S.; Dandona, L. Patterns of road traffic injuries in a vulnerable population in Hyderabad. *India Inj. Prev.* **2006**, *12*, 183–188. [CrossRef] [PubMed]

39. Seid, M.; Azazh, A.; Enquselassie, F.; Yisma, E. Injury characteristics and outcome of road traffic accident among victims at Adult Emergency Department of Tikur Anbessa specialized hospital, Addis Ababa, Ethiopia: A prospective hospital based study. *BMC Emerg. Med.* **2015**, *15*, 10. [CrossRef] [PubMed]

40. Datta, S.K.; Tanushree, D. Rural poverty and female job participation: A case study of two districts in West Bengal. *Bangladesh Dev. Stud.* **2015**, *38*, 55–76.

41. Giashuddin, S.M.; Rahman, A.; Rahman, F.; Mashreky, S.R.; Chowdhury, S.M.; Linnan, M.; Shafinaz, S. Socioeconomic inequality in child injury in Bangladesh–implication for developing countries. *Int. J. Equity Health* **2009**, *8*, 7. [CrossRef] [PubMed]

42. Christie, N. The High-Risk Child Pedestrian: Socio-Economic and Environmental Factors in Their Accidents. TRL Project Report. 1995. Available online: https://trid.trb.org/view.aspx?id=451297 (accessed on 7 September 2016).

43. World Health Organization. Road Traffic Injuries, Fact Sheet, Updated May 2017. Available online: http://www.who.int/mediacentre/factsheets/fs358/en/ (accessed on 9 June 2017).

44. Ghimire, A.; Nagesh, S.; Jha, N.; Niraula, S.R.; Devkota, S. An epidemiological study of injury among urban population. *Kathmandu Univ. Med. J.* **2009**, *7*, 402–407. [CrossRef]

45. Moe, H. Road traffic injuries among patients who attended the accident and emergency unit of the University of Malaya medical centre of the University of Malaya medical centre, Kuala Lumpur. *J. Univ. Malaya Med. Cent. (JUMMEC)* **2008**, *11*, 22–26.

46. Biswas, A.; Kibria, A.; Hossain, S.T.; Rahman, F.; Baset, K.U.; Mashreky, S.R. A seat belt in non-motorised vehicle rickshaw—can it prevent roads traffic injuries in Bangladesh? *Inj. Prev.* **2012**, *18* (Suppl. 1), A199. [CrossRef]

47. Rab, M.A. Rural Road Safety Problem and Prospects in Bangladesh Context. In Proceedings of the International Conference on Road Safety in Developing Countries, Dhaka, Bangladesh, 22–24 August 2006; Accident Research Centre, BUET: Melbourne, Victoria, Australia, 2006.

48. Nantulya, V.M.; Reich, M.R. The neglected epidemic: Road traffic injuries in developing countries. *BMJ Br. Med. J.* **2002**, *324*, 1139. [CrossRef]

49. Afukaar, F.K.; Antwi, P.; Ofosu-Amaah, S. Pattern of road traffic injuries in Ghana: Implications for control. *Inj. Control Saf. Promot.* **2003**, *10*, 69–76. [CrossRef] [PubMed]

50. Nantulya, V.M.; Reich, M.R. Equity dimensions of road traffic injuries in low-and middle-income countries. *Inj. Control Saf. Promot.* **2003**, *10*, 13–20. [CrossRef] [PubMed]

51. Van der Horst, A.R.; Thierry, M.C.; Vet, J.M.; Rahman, A.F. An evaluation of speed management measures in Bangladesh based upon alternative accident recording, speed measurements, and DOCTOR traffic conflict observations. *Transp. Res. Part F Traffic Psychol. Behav.* **2017**, *46*, 390–403. [CrossRef]

52. Transport Notes. *Notes on the Economic Evaluation of Transport Projects*; Transport Note No. TRN-21; Transport Economics, Policy and Poverty Thematic Group, The World Bank: Washington, DC, USA, January 2005. Available online: http://siteresources.worldbank.org/INTTRANSPORT/Resources/336291-1227561426235/5611053-1231943010251/trn-21EENote2.pdf (accessed on 2 July 2016).

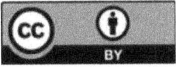

International Journal of
*Environmental Research
and Public Health*

MDPI

Article

Epidemiology of Fall Injury in Rural Bangladesh

Shirin Wadhwaniya [1],*, Olakunle Alonge [1], Md. Kamran Ul Baset [2], Salim Chowdhury [2],
Al-Amin Bhuiyan [2] and Adnan A. Hyder [1]

[1]   Johns Hopkins International Injury Research Unit, Department of International Health, Johns Hopkins
      Bloomberg School of Public Health, 615 N. Wolfe Street, Baltimore, MD 21205, USA;
      oalonge1@jhu.edu (O.A.); ahyder1@jhu.edu (A.A.H)
[2]   Center for Injury Prevention and Research, Bangladesh (CIPRB), House B162, Road 23, New DOHS,
      Mohakhali, Dhaka 1206, Bangladesh; kamran_baset@yahoo.co.uk (M.K.U.B.);
      smchow_dhaka@yahoo.com (S.C.); al-amin@ciprb.org (A.-A.B.)
*   Correspondence: swadhwa2@jhu.edu

Academic Editor: David C. Schwebel
Received: 6 June 2017; Accepted: 3 August 2017; Published: 10 August 2017

Abstract: Globally, falls are the second leading cause of unintentional injury deaths, with 80%
occurring in low-and middle-income countries. The overall objective of this study is to describe
the burden and risk factors of falls in rural Bangladesh. In 2013, a large household survey covering
a population of 1,169,593 was conducted in seven rural sub-districts of Bangladesh to assess the
burden of all injuries, including falls. The recall periods for non-fatal and fatal injuries were six
and 12 months, respectively. Descriptive, bivariate and multiple logistic regression analyses were
conducted. The rates of non-fatal and fatal falls were 36.3 per 1000 and 5 per 100,000 population,
respectively. The rates of both fatal and non-fatal falls were highest among the elderly. The risk of
non-fatal falls was higher at extremes of age. Lower limb and waist injuries were frequent following
a fall. Head injuries were frequent among infants (35%), while lower limb and waist injuries were
frequent among the elderly (>65 years old). Injuries to all body parts (except the waist) were most
frequent among men. More than half of all non-fatal falls occurred in a home environment. The injury
patterns and risk factors of non-fatal falls differ by sociodemographic factors.

Keywords: injury; fall injury; Bangladesh; LMICs

1. Introduction

Annually, about 4.7 million deaths are due to injury, and these account for about 8.5% of the global
disease burden [1]. The majority (80%) of these deaths occur in low-and middle-income countries
(LMICs) and the World Health Organization's South-East Asia region has the highest unintentional
injury mortality rate (80 per 100,000) and the highest rate for disability-adjusted life years (DALYs)
due to unintentional injuries (3065 per 100,000) in the world [2,3]. Falls are the second leading cause of
unintentional injury deaths, and the 13th leading cause of global years lived with disability (YLD) [1–4].
Between 2005–2015, global deaths due to fall increased by about 21%, and a major contributor for this
was population growth and aging [1]. If left unaddressed, the burden of fall injuries is projected to
increase by 100% by the year 2030 [5].

Fall can occur on the same level as a result of slipping or tripping, or at a different level, such as a
fall from a height [2,5]. Several sociodemographic, occupational, health or medical, and environmental
factors have been identified as risk factors for falls [2,5]. Globally, the burden of fall injuries is higher
among the elderly (>65 years), and this burden increases with age [5]. However, children are also
vulnerable to falls [6,7]. There is limited epidemiological data on fall injuries in LMICs [5].

Bangladesh, a lower-middle income country in the South Asia, has a high burden of disability as
a result of injury, including falls [8]. Previous studies from Bangladesh have reported a high burden of

fall-related mortality, morbidity and disability among children [9–11]. The government of Bangladesh has recognized injury prevention as a national priority [8]. However, most fall injury-related studies from Bangladesh have focused on specific population or group. An in-depth population-based study on the epidemiology of falls can provide information on risk factors and would help in planning effective prevention strategies. The overall goals of this study are to describe the burden of fall injuries, identify risk factors and patterns of fall injuries, and make recommendations to reduce the burden of falls in rural Bangladesh.

2. Materials and Methods

As part of the Saving of Lives from Drowning (SoLiD) project, a large baseline survey was conducted from June–November 2013 in seven purposively selected sub-districts—Matlab North, Matlab South, Daudkandi, Chandpur Sadar, Raiganj, Sherpur Sadar and Manohardi—covering a population of approximately 1.16 million people in 51 unions [12,13]. The data collection method for this survey has been described earlier, and is summarized below [14].

All data collectors received training on research methods, data collection tools, and ethics. Prior to starting with data collection, mapping and household listing was conducted in all villages. During this exercise, each household was assigned a serial number based on a predetermined format. All households in the selected sub-district were visited i.e., a census survey was conducted. A written consent was obtained prior to starting data collection. Data was collected from either the head of the household or any adult member of the household aged 18 years and older. Household, sociodemographic and injury data were collected for all individuals in each household. The birth history of all ever-married women who were between 15–49 years of age was obtained. Data on all injury mortality and morbidity were collected. Injury mortality data was collected over a 12-month recall period, while injury morbidity data was collected over a six-month recall period. Only injuries for which care was sought from either a formal or informal provider, and/or there was loss of work/daily activities for a day, were included in the survey.

Household, sociodemographic data and birth history were collected by one set of data collectors, who were also responsible for completing an injury notification form for any injury mortality and morbidity event that occurred during the recall period. Based on the outcomes recorded on the injury notification form, a second set of data collectors visited households to complete injury mortality/morbidity and mechanism forms. All of the forms were developed in English, translated to Bangla, and then back-translated and pilot-tested prior to data collection.

A dichotomous variable for fall injury—yes or no—was created. In case of multiple falls, only one event per person was taken into consideration for analysis. Sub-district, age group, sex, education, marital status and occupation were categorical variables. Using principle component analysis, households were categorized into five quintiles: lowest, low, middle, high, and highest. Rates for fall-related mortality and morbidity by each category were calculated. These are expressed per 100,000 and per 1000 population for mortality and morbidity, respectively.

Simple descriptive analysis and bivariate cross-tabulations were conducted [15]. To explore differences in fall-related mortality and morbidity by sociodemographic categories, the Chi-square test or Fisher's exact test (when conditions for Chi-square were violated) were conducted [15]. For both fall mortality and morbidity, bivariate logistic regression analyses were used to study the association of each covariate with fall mortality and morbidity [15]. These covariates included sub-district, age group, sex, education, marital status, occupation, and socioeconomic status. Multivariate logistic regressions (MLR) were performed for fall morbidity using the same explanatory variables [15]. For non-fatal falls, a comparison of results from bivariate and MLR indicated an interaction between age and sex; hence, another model with an interaction term including age group and sex was run. The multivariate models without and with the interaction term were compared using the likelihood ratio test and the model with the interaction term was significant (<0.001). For fatal falls; age, education, marital status and occupation groups were re-categorized, as there were no fall-related deaths in some groups. To address the separation issue, Firth logit regression was run for fatal falls. In the Firth logit regression model; sub-district, age group, sex, education, marital status, occupation, and socioeconomic status were included as covariates. Injured body parts were combined into seven body regions: head and neck, face, chest, abdomen, upper limb, lower limb, and waist. The proportion of fall cases that had injury to a particular body region by age group and sex were calculated.

All analyses were carried out using STATA version 12 and 13 (StataCorp LP, College Station, Texas, USA), and $p < 0.05$ was considered statistically significant [16]. The Institutional Review Board of the Johns Hopkins Bloomberg School of Public Health (JHSPH), and the Ethics Review Committees of the International Center for Diarrhoeal Disease Research, Bangladesh (icddr, b), and Center for Injury Prevention and Research, Bangladesh (CIPRB), approved this study (JHSPH IRB 00004746).

3. Results

The baseline survey covered a total of 1,169,593 individuals in seven rural sub-districts of Bangladesh. About 39% of the population was children (<18 years), and about 55% were in the productive age group (18–64 years). The overall male to female ratio was 1:1.06. Nearly a quarter of the population did not have any formal education, and nearly half were married. About 35% were either retired, unemployed, or housewives. The distribution of the population in five wealth quintiles was nearly equal (Table 1).

Table 1. Sociodemographic characteristics of fatal and non-fatal fall injury patients in rural Bangladesh.

	Fatal Fall Injury (*N* = 59)			Non-Fatal Fall Injury (*N* = 42,259)			Total (*N* = 1,169,593)
	N	Rate Per 100,000 Population (95% CI)	*p* Value	*N*	Rate Per 1000 Population (95% CI)	*p* Value	*N* (%)
Sub-district							
Matlab North	21	7.9 (4.5–11.3)		12,058	45.6 (44.8–46.4)		265,897 (22.7)
Matlab South	15	7.2 (3.5–10.8)		11,435	54.8 (53.8–55.8)		209,772 (17.9)
Chandpur Sadar	3	2.3 (0.0–5.0)		4570	35.8 (34.8–36.8)		128,356 (11.0)
Raiganj	2	1.9 (0.0–4.6)	0.030 *	3554	34.3 (33.1–35.4)	<0.001 ***	104,357 (8.9)
Sherpur Sadar	8	3.5 (1.1–5.9)		4059	17.9 (17.3–18.4)		228,519 (19.5)
Manohardi	7	3.4 (0.9–6.0)		4680	23.0 (22.4–23.7)		204,319 (17.5)
Daudkandi	3	10.6 (0.0–22.5)		1903	67.5 (64.6–70.5)		28,373 (2.4)
Age group							
<1 year	0	-		280	13.0 (11.5–14.5)		22,141 (1.9)
1–4 years	0	-		2927	32.5 (31.3–33.6)		90,523 (7.7)
5–9 years	3	2.2 (0.0–4.6)		4453	31.9 (31.0–32.8)		139,728 (12.0)
10–14 years	1	0.7 (0.0–2.1)		3848	27.1 (26.2–27.9)		142,121 (12.2)
15–17 years	0	-	-	1435	23.1 (21.9–24.3)	<0.001 ***	62,098 (5.3)
18–24 years	2	1.5 (0.0–3.6)		2879	21.6 (20.8–22.4)		133,534 (11.4)
25–64 years	14	2.8 (1.3–4.2)		22,273	44.0 (43.4–44.6)		508,059 (43.4)
>64 years	39	54.6 (37.5–71.8)		4164	61.0 (59.2–62.8)		71,389 (6.1)
Sex							
Male	31	5.5 (3.5–7.4)	0.538	18,312	32.4 (32.0–32.9)	<0.001 ***	567,674 (48.5)
Female	28	4.7 (2.9–6.4)		23,947	40.0 (39.5–40.5)		601,919 (51.5)
Education							
No education	39	13.2 (9.1–17.4)		12,608	43.2 (42.5–43.9)		295,314 (25.3)
Primary	10	2.5 (0.9–4.0)		15,734	38.7 (38.1–39.2)		407,923 (34.9)
Secondary	8	2.8 (0.8–4.7)		9228	31.9 (31.3–32.6)		289,658 (24.8)
A levels	1	2.2 (0.0–6.5)	<0.001 ***	1079	23.7 (22.3–25.1)	<0.001 ***	45,618 (3.9)
College	0	-		299	22.2 (19.7–24.7)		13,526 (1.2)
Advanced/Professional degree	0	-		100	21.3 (17.2–25.4)		4729 (0.4)
Not applicable (under 5 children)	0	-		3207	28.7 (27.7–29.7)		112,664 (9.6)
Marital status							
Married	33	5.8 (3.8–7.8)		23,845	42.0 (41.5–42.5)		571,206 (48.8)
Never married	2	0.9 (0.0–2.1)		5052	22.2 (21.6–22.9)		227,319 (19.4)
Divorced	0	-		116	36.3 (29.8–42.8)		3220 (0.3)
Widowed	20	37.7 (21.2–54.2)	<0.001 ***	3695	71.6 (69.3–73.8)	<0.001 ***	53,096 (4.5)
Separated	0	-		128	47.4 (39.4–55.4)		2717 (0.2)
Not applicable	4	1.3 (0.0–2.5)		9423	30.3 (29.7–30.9)		312,035 (26.7)

Table 1. *Cont.*

	Fatal Fall Injury (*N* = 59)			Non-Fatal Fall Injury (*N* = 42,259)			Total (*N* = 1,169,593)
	N	Rate Per 100,000 Population (95% CI)	*p* Value	*N*	Rate Per 1000 Population (95% CI)	*p* Value	*N* (%)
Occupation							
Agriculture	9	8.6 (3.0–14.2)		3440	33.1 (32.1–34.2)		104,956 (9.0)
Business	3	4.9 (0.0–10.4)		1518	24.8 (23.5–26.0)		61,661 (5.3)
Skilled labor (Professional)	5	5.6 (0.7–10.5)		2250	25.3 (24.3–26.4)		89,151 (7.6)
Unskilled/domestic labor	0	-	-	894	36.6 (34.3–39.0)	<0.001 ***	24,520 (2.1)
Rickshaw/bus (transport worker)	1	5.9 (0.0–17.4)		445	26.2 (23.8–28.6)		17,037 (1.5)
Students	3	1.0 (0.0–2.1)		8580	27.5 (26.9–28.0)		312,537 (26.7)
Retired/unemployed/housewife	36	8.8 (5.9–11.7)		20,716	51.1 (50.4–51.7)		408,583 (34.9)
Not applicable (children)	0	-		4195	29.3 (28.4–30.1)		144,454 (12.4)
Not applicable (others)	2	33.6 (0.0–80.2)		195	33.7 (29.1–38.4)		5948 (0.5)
Socioeconomic status							
Lowest	7	3.3 (0.9–5.8)		7714	36.7 (35.9–37.5)		211,601 (18.1)
Low	11	5.0 (2.1–8.0)		7927	36.4 (35.6–37.2)		218,695 (18.7)
Middle	11	4.6 (1.9–7.3)	0.653	9051	38.2 (37.4–39.0)	<0.001 ***	238,371 (20.4)
High	16	6.5 (3.3–9.6)		9051	36.7 (36.0–37.4)		247,716 (21.2)
Highest	14	5.5 (2.6–8.4)		8516	33.8 (33.1–34.5)		253,201 (21.7)

Missing: education for 0.01% (n = 151), occupation for 0.06% (n = 737); *** $p < 0.001$, * $p < 0.05$.

3.1. Fatal Fall Injury

A total 59 fatal falls were recorded in the survey, and the mortality rate in this population was 5 per 100,000 persons (Table 1). Fall mortality rates were highest in the Daudkandi sub-district (10.6 per 100,000 population). Nearly 66% of fatal falls were among the elderly (those above the age of 64 years), with a mortality rate of 54.6 per 100,000 population. Fall mortality rates were also higher among those with no formal education, and among the widowed (Table 1).

3.2. Non-Fatal Fall Injury

Of the total 1,169,593 individuals who were surveyed, 42,259 reported to have experienced at least one fall injury in the six months preceding the survey. The incidence of non-fatal fall in this population was 36.3 per 1000 population. Fall morbidity rates were highest in the Daudkandi sub-district (67.5 per 1000 population), and among those above the age of 64 years (61 per 1000 population). Nearly 57% of falls were among women. Rates of non-fatal falls were also higher among those with no formal education, the widowed, the retired or unemployed, and housewives (Table 1).

Lower limb (42.5%), upper limb (25.5%), and waist (29.6%) were the most common body regions injured in a fall. A statistically significant association was found between injured body parts and age and sex. Head, face and chest injuries were frequent in younger children (<4 years); upper limb injuries were frequent in older children (5–9 years old); lower limb injuries were frequent in young adults (10–24 years old); and waist injuries were frequent in adults over 24 years of age (Figure 1a). Men more frequently injured all the listed body regions, with the exception of the waist ($p < 0.001$, Figure 1b).

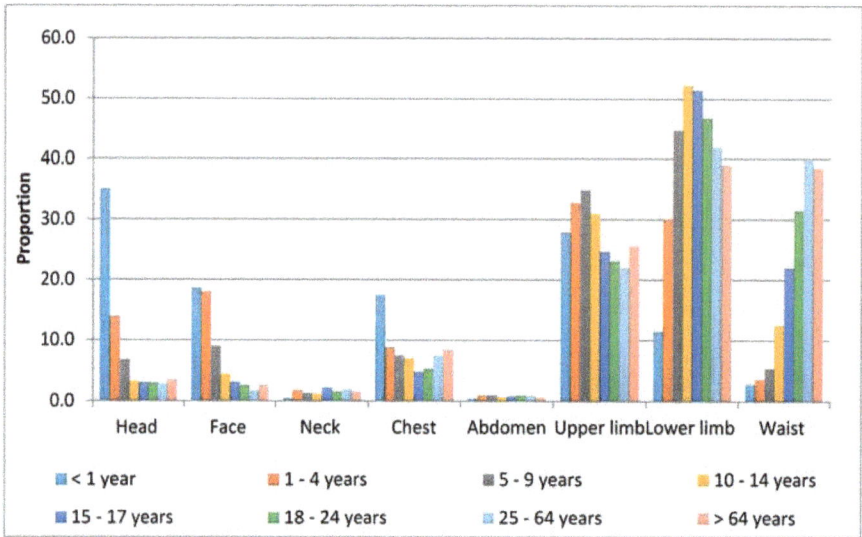

p value < 0.001 for head, face, chest, upper limb, lower limb, and waist; p value < 0.01 for neck

(a)

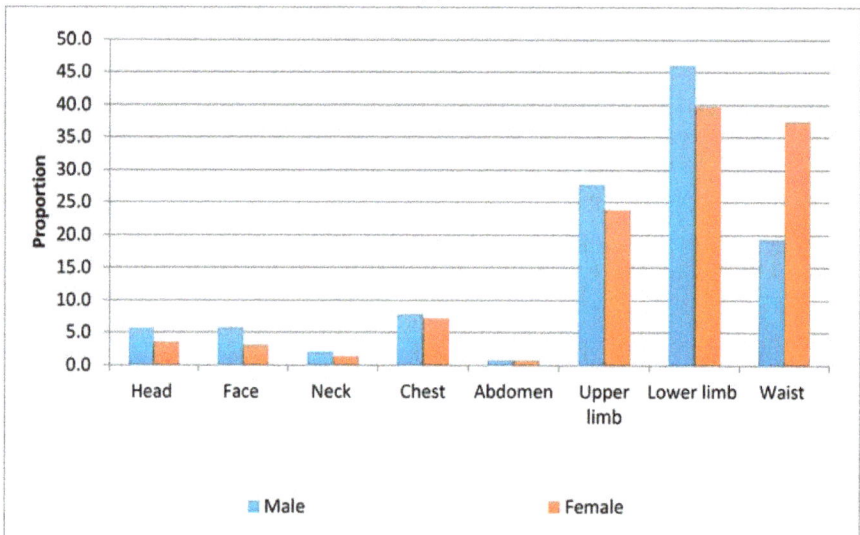

p value < 0.001 for head, face, neck, upper limb, hand, and lower limb waist

(b)

Figure 1. Body parts injured in non-fatal falls by age groups and sex. (**a**) Injured body parts by age groups; (**b**) Injured body parts by sex.

The majority (70%) of falls were at the same level, and most falls occurred in either external or internal home environments. Most falls among women were within a home environment, while the majority of falls among men were outside the home (Figure 2a). The majority of falls among children <4 years and adults (>18 years) were also in either internal or external home environments, while most falls among adolescents were outside the home (Figure 2b).

(a)

(b)

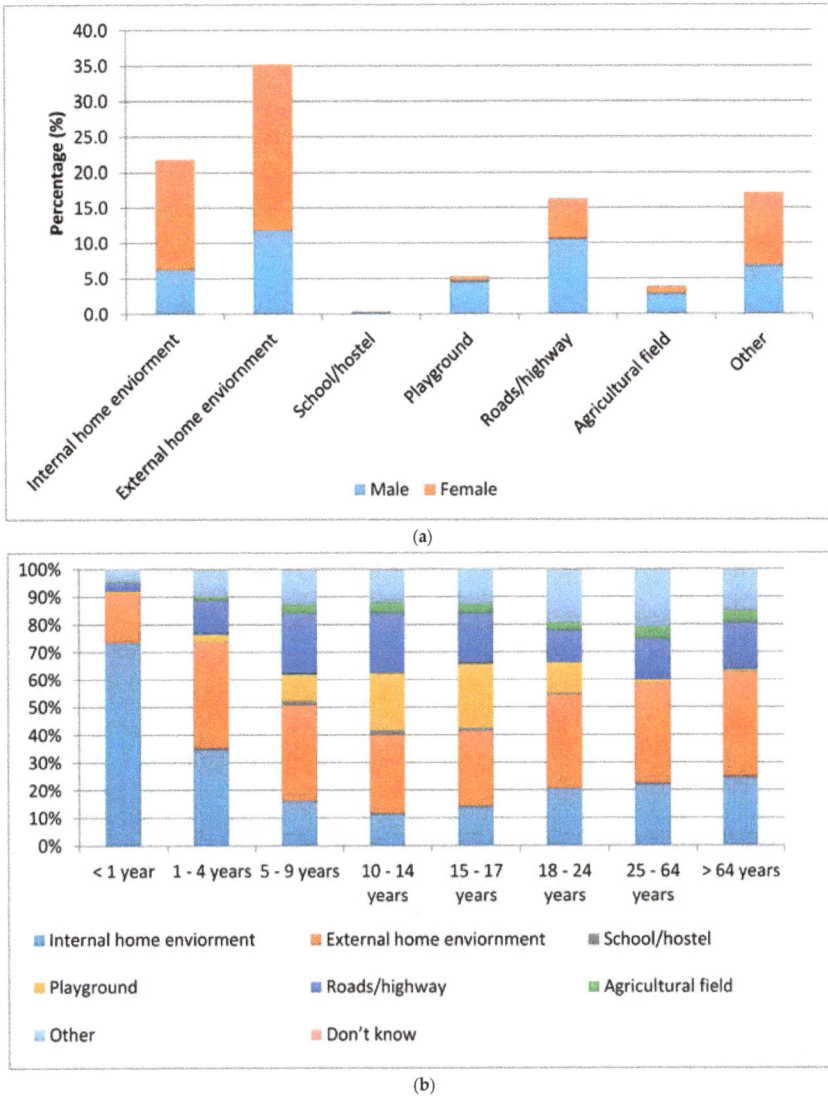

Figure 2. Place of non-fatal fall injuries by sex and age. (**a**) Place of injury by sex; (**b**) Place of injury by age group.

Nearly 70% of all falls had occurred at the same level as a result of slipping/tripping (66%) or stumbling (26%). Also, most of the same-level falls occurred on a sidewalk or street (62%), followed by within the home environment (18%), while most of the different-level falls were from a tree (27%), stairs (25%), or furniture (18%).

3.3. Factors Associated with Fatal Falls

Compared to children (<18 years), the elderly (>64 years) had higher odds of experiencing fatal falls. Education played a protective role for fall injury; those with any education were 70% less likely to sustain fatal falls compared with those with no formal education (Table 2). Individuals who were divorced, widowed, or separated had nearly six times higher odds of suffering fatal falls compared with those who were married. No statistically significant association was found between fatal falls and sub-district. No significant difference was found between fatal falls and socioeconomic status (Table 2).

Table 2. Factors associated with fatal fall injuries in Bangladesh.

	Unadjusted		Adjusted ^	
	Odds Ratio (95% CI)	*p* Value	Odds Ratio (95% CI)	*p* Value
Sub-district				
Matlab North	1	-	1	-
Matlab South	0.9 (0.5–1.8)	0.769	1.0 (0.5–1.9)	0.976
Chandpur Sadar	0.3 (0.1–1.0)	0.049 *	0.4 (0.1–1.2)	0.111
Raiganj	0.2 (0.1–1.0)	0.056	0.3 (0.1–1.2)	0.098
Sherpur Sadar	0.4 (0.2–1.0)	0.050	0.6 (0.3–1.4)	0.229
Manohardi	0.4 (0.2–1.0)	0.056	0.5 (0.2–1.2)	0.123
Daudkandi	1.3 (0.4–4.5)	0.636	1.4 (0.4–4.3)	0.567
Age group				
<18 years	1	-	1	-
18–24 years	1.7 (0.3–9.3)	0.536	5.0 (0.1–333.1)	0.456
25–64 years	3.1 (1.0–9.6)	0.043 *	5.9 (0.1–500.6)	0.431
>64 years	62.4 (22.3–174.6)	<0.001 ***	71.7 (0.8–6285.6)	0.061
Sex				
Male	1	-	1	-
Female	0.9 (0.5–1.4)	0.538	0.5 (0.3–1.1)	0.107
Education				
No education (includes under 5 children)	1	-	1	-
Primary	0.3 (0.1–0.5)	<0.001 ***	0.4 (0.2–0.9)	0.023 *
Secondary and higher	0.3 (0.1–0.5)	<0.001 ***	0.5 (0.2–1.1)	0.099
Marital status				
Married	1	-	1	-
Never married	0.2 (0.0–0.6)	0.010 **	1.5 (0.3–8.3)	0.655
Divorced/widowed/separated	5.9 (3.4–10.2)	<0.001 ***	2.1 (1.0–4.3)	0.053
Not applicable	0.2 (0.1–0.6)	0.004 **	11.1 (0.1–996.8)	0.294
Occupation				
Agriculture	1	-	1	-
Business	0.6 (0.2–2.1)	0.395	1.2 (0.3–4.2)	0.784
Skilled labor (Professional)	0.7 (0.2–2.0)	0.447	1.8 (0.6–5.7)	0.291
Unskilled/semi-skilled labor	0.3 (0.0–2.2)	0.228	0.8 (0.1–4.5)	0.779
Students	0.1 (0.0–0.4)	0.001 **	0.5 (0.0–5.7)	0.598
Retired/unemployed/housewife	1.0 (0.5–2.1)	0.942	1.1 (0.4–2.7)	0.843
Not applicable	0.2 (0.0–0.7)	0.017 *	0.1 (0.0–1.9)	0.138
Socioeconomic status				
Lowest	1		1	
Low	1.5 (0.6–3.9)	0.386	1.6 (0.6–4.2)	0.303
Middle	1.4 (0.5–3.6)	0.491	1.5 (0.6–3.9)	0.362
High	2.0 (0.8–4.7)	0.140	2.1 (0.9–5.2)	0.094
Highest	1.7 (0.7–4.1)	0.267	1.8 (0.7–4.6)	0.203

*** $p < 0.001$, ** $p < 0.01$, * $p < 0.05$, ^ firthlogit regression.

After adjusting for other covariates, no significant relationship was found between fatal falls and sub-district, age group, sex, marital status, occupation, or socioeconomic status (Table 2). Those with primary education were 60% less likely to experience fatal falls compared with those with no formal education.

3.4. Factors Associated with Non-Fatal Falls

Compared to Matlab North, the populations in Daudkandi and Matlab South had higher odds of sustaining non-fatal falls. The odds of experiencing non-fatal falls show a bimodal distribution by age group. After infancy, the odds increase for 1–4-year-olds, it then plateaus between the ages of 10 and 24 years, and then increases again among those above 24 years of age (Table 3). Women were 1.2 times likely to sustain non-fatal falls, compared with men. The odds of experiencing fall injury were highest among those with no formal education, and the odds reduced with increasing education level ($p < 0.001$, Table 3).

The widowed had 1.8 times higher odds of having non-fatal falls ($p < 0.001$) compared with married individuals. Also, compared with those involved in agriculture, the odds of experiencing falls were 1.6 times higher among the retired, the unemployed, and housewives (Table 3). Compared with those in the lowest socioeconomic status (SES) group, those in the highest SES group had a 10% lower risk of sustaining falls ($p < 0.001$). The relationship between non-fatal falls and the middle SES group was statistically significant, but not meaningful (Table 3).

Table 3. Factors associated with non-fatal fall injuries in Bangladesh.

	Unadjusted		Adjusted #	
	Odds Ratio (95% CI)	*p* Value	Odds Ratio (95% CI)	*p* Value
Sub-district				
Matlab North	1	-	1	-
Matlab South	1.2 (1.2–1.2)	<0.001 ***	1.2 (1.2–1.3)	<0.001 ***
Chandpur Sadar	0.8 (0.8–0.8)	<0.001 ***	0.8 (0.8–0.8)	<0.001 ***
Raiganj	0.7 (0.7–0.8)	<0.001 ***	0.7 (0.7–0.8)	<0.001 ***
Sherpur Sadar	0.4 (0.4–0.4)	<0.001 ***	0.4 (0.4–0.4)	<0.001 ***
Manohardi	0.5 (0.5–0.5)	<0.001 ***	0.5 (0.5–0.5)	<0.001 ***
Daudkandi	1.5 (1.4–1.6)	<0.001 ***	1.5 (1.4–1.6)	<0.001 ***
Age group				
<1 year	1	-	1	-
1–4 years	2.5 (2.3–2.9)	<0.001 ***	2.9 (2.4–3.4)	<0.001 ***
5–9 years	2.5 (2.2–2.8)	<0.001 ***	1.1 (0.9–1.2)	0.349
10–14 years	2.1 (1.9–2.4)	<0.001 ***	1.0 (0.9–1.1)	0.640
15–17 years	1.8 (1.6–2.0)	<0.001 ***	0.9 (0.8–1.0)	0.012 *
18–24 years	1.7 (1.5–1.9)	<0.001 ***	0.7 (0.6–0.8)	<0.001 ***
25–64 years	3.5 (3.1–3.9)	<0.001 ***	0.8 (0.7–0.8)	<0.001 ***
> 64 years	4.9 (4.4–5.6)	<0.001 ***	-	-
Sex				
Male	1	-	1	-
Female	1.2 (1.2–1.3)	<0.001 ***	0.9 (0.7–1.2)	0.550
Education				
No education	1	-	1	-
Primary	0.9 (0.9–0.9)	<0.001 ***	1.1 (1.0–1.1)	<0.001 ***
Secondary	0.7 (0.7–0.8)	<0.001 ***	0.9 (0.9–0.9)	<0.001 ***
A levels	0.5 (0.5–0.6)	<0.001 ***	0.8 (0.7–0.8)	<0.001 ***
College	0.5 (0.4–0.6)	<0.001 ***	0.7 (0.6–0.8)	<0.001 ***
Advanced/Professional degree	0.5 (0.4–0.6)	<0.001 ***	0.6 (0.5–0.8)	<0.001 ***
Not applicable (under 5 children)	0.7 (0.6–0.7)	<0.001 ***	0.3 (0.3–0.4)	<0.001 ***
Marital status				
Married	1	-	1	-
Never married	0.5 (0.5–0.5)	<0.001 ***	0.6 (0.6–0.7)	<0.001 ***
Divorced	0.9 (0.7–1.0)	0.108	0.9 (0.7–1.0)	0.115
Widowed	1.8 (1.7–1.8)	<0.001 ***	1.2 (1.2–1.3)	<0.001 ***
Separated	1.1 (0.9–1.4)	0.165	1.1 (0.9–1.3)	0.302
Not applicable	0.7 (0.7–0.7)	<0.001 ***	0.7 (0.6–0.7)	<0.001 ***
Occupation				
Agriculture	1	-	1	-
Business	0.7 (0.7–0.8)	<0.001 ***	0.7 (0.7–0.8)	<0.001 ***
Skilled labor (Professional)	0.8 (0.7–0.8)	<0.001 ***	0.8 (0.8–0.8)	<0.001 ***
Unskilled/domestic labor	1.1 (1.0–1.2)	0.006 **	1.1 (1.0–1.2)	0.029 *
Rickshaw/bus (transport worker)	0.8 (0.7–0.9)	<0.001 ***	0.8 (0.7–0.9)	<0.001 ***
Students	0.8 (0.8–0.9)	<0.001 ***	1.2 (1.1–1.3)	<0.001 ***
Retired/unemployed/housewife	1.6 (1.5–1.6)	<0.001 ***	1.1 (1.0–1.1)	0.079
Not applicable (children)	0.9 (0.8–0.9)	<0.001 ***	1.2 (1.1–1.3)	0.001 **
Not applicable (others)	1.0 (0.9–0.2)	0.807	1.3 (1.1–1.5)	0.002 **
Socioeconomic status				
Lowest	1	-	1	-
Low	1.0 (1.0–1.0)	0.650	1.0 (0.9–1.0)	0.145
Middle	1.0 (1.0–1.1)	0.009 **	1.0 (0.9–1.0)	0.043 *
High	1.0 (1.0–1.0)	0.942	1.0 (0.9–1.0)	0.002 *
Highest	0.9 (0.9–0.9)	<0.001 ***	0.9 (0.9–0.9)	<0.001 ***

Adjusted for Age group and sex interaction; *** $p < 0.001$, ** $p < 0.01$, * $p < 0.05$.

After controlling for age, sex, education, marital status, occupation, socioeconomic status, and introducing the age–sex interaction terms; the odds of sustaining non-fatal falls for different sub-districts remained significant. The odds of fall injury were 2.9 times higher among 1–4-year-olds compared with infants. After adjusting for other covariates, the relationship between sex and non-fatal falls did not remain significant. However, even after adjusting, those widowed continued to have higher odds of sustaining falls compared with their reference group (Table 3). The odds of having fall injuries were also significantly higher among the unskilled and domestic laborers, students, and children, compared with those involved in agricultural work (Table 3).

Female infants were 90% less likely to sustain falls compared with male infants ($p < 0.001$, Table 4). Among 1–4-year-olds, females were 2.7 times more likely to experience falls compared with 1–4-year-old males ($p < 0.001$, Table 4). However, 18–64-year-old females were 30% less likely to sustain falls compared with men in the same age category (Table 4).

Table 4. Adjusted odds of fall injuries by age and sex.

	Odds Ratio (95% CI)	*p*-Value
<1 year female compared to <1 year male	0.1 (0.0–0.1)	<0.001 ***
1–4 years female compared to 1–4 years male	2.7 (1.9–3.9)	<0.001 ***
5–9 years female compared to 5–9 years male	1.0 (0.8–1.3)	0.894
10–14 years female compared to 10–14 years male	1.0 (0.7–1.2)	0.710
15–17 years female compared to 15–17 years male	0.8 (0.6–1.1)	0.115
18–24 years female compared to 18–24 years male	0.7 (0.5–0.8)	0.001 **
25–64 years female compared to 25–64 years male	0.7 (0.6–0.9)	0.006 **
>65 years female compared to >65 years male	0.9 (0.7–1.2)	0.550

*** $p < 0.001$, ** $p < 0.01$.

4. Discussion

To our knowledge, this is the first study describing the epidemiology of fall injuries among the general population in Bangladesh. Previous studies from Bangladesh have either focused on specific segments of the population or groups [9,10,17,18]. The rates of fatal and non-fatal falls were 5 per 100,000 population, and 36.3 per 1000 population, respectively. The rates of fatal and non-fatal falls were highest among the elderly. Other groups vulnerable to non-fatal falls included children, the widowed, unskilled/domestic laborers, and students. Residents of Matlab South and Daudkandi were also vulnerable for falls, while those in the highest SES group had a lower risk.

In our study, about 66% of all fatal falls were among the elderly. Falling can lead to physical disability, but it may also affect the mental, social and emotional well-being of the elderly [5]. In the last decade, Bangladesh has made significant achievements to improve health indicators, and the life expectancy at birth has also increased from 67.5 in 2004 to 71.6 years in 2014 [19]. With the increase in the aging population, the burden of fall injuries is also expected to increase in LMICs, including Bangladesh, and there is a need to focus on interventions that prevent falls among this age group [5,20].

In high-income settings, primary prevention interventions that promote physical activity and healthy lifestyles among the elderly have been implemented to prevent fall injuries [5,21]. Interventions for fall risk assessment and management are also found to be effective [21]. These programs may focus on the management of medications and health problems related to vision, foot, orthostatic hypotension, cardiovascular problems, gait, and balance [5]. Environmental modifications at home and within communities are also recommended [5]. Secondary prevention strategies such as the use of hip protectors to prevent hip fracture in the event of a fall have also been implemented [2,5]. Tertiary prevention strategies may focus on rehabilitation and improvement of functions to prevent disability following a fall. [5] However, there is a dearth of effective fall-prevention interventions from LMICs, including Bangladesh, and there is limited evidence on the acceptability of these interventions in this setting [20,22,23].

Children emerged as the other vulnerable group for fall injuries. Earlier studies from LMICs and Bangladesh have also highlighted this [6,7,10,17,18,24,25]. A multisite unintentional injury surveillance study conducted in five LMICs found that about half of all emergency department visits among children aged 0–12 years were as a result of falls [7]. Again, most fall injuries are found to occur in or around the home environment, and during play [6,7,10,17,18]. This could be because children in LMICs lack designated and safe play areas [26]. Strategies such as installing window guards, making environmental modifications in and around homes, and enforcing standards in playgrounds may also help prevent fall injuries among children [4].

Globally, elderly women are more likely to suffer from fall injuries compared with men [4]. However, no gender difference in the distribution of fatal and non-fatal falls among the elderly was found in this study. In our study, men in the productive age group (18–64 years) had a higher risk of falling compared with women in the same age category. In rural Bangladesh, men play an active role outside the home, and may be involved in high-risk behaviors and occupations that increase their risk of falling [2]. Previous studies have found falls to be more frequent among boys [6,7,10,17,18]. This could be because boys tend to play outside the house, and are exposed to greater risk compared with girls, who are mostly involved in household activities [17,18]. Contrary to earlier findings, in our study, 1–4-year-old girls had a relatively higher risk of sustaining non-fatal falls compared with boys in the same age group. Further research is required to explain the gender difference in this age group.

In this study, falls among young children, women, and the elderly were more frequent within the home environment, while those among men and adolescents were more frequently outside. In Bangladesh, children, women, and the elderly tend to spend more time at home, and this can explain the higher incidence of falls within the home environment for these groups. In contrast, men and adolescents spend more time outside the home, and this can explain the higher incidence of falls outside the home environment [27].

Our study found a higher risk of fall injuries among the widowed. This could be because these individuals are more likely to live alone, lack social support, have lower income, and experience physical and mental health problems that increase their risk of falls [5]. In our study, we found that compared to those in the lowest SES group, those in the highest SES category had a slightly lower risk of falls. This may be due to differences in the designs and materials used for constructing houses amongst SES groups; the housing structure of the highest SES group may be safer and less injury-prone compared with those in the lowest SES category.

In our study, the pattern and the distribution of injuries resulting from falls varied by age and sex. Young children were more likely to suffer from head and chest injuries; older children and adolescents were more likely to suffer from limb injuries; while young adults and the elderly were more likely to suffer from lower limb and waist injuries. These findings are comparable with those found in other studies [27,28].

The risk of falls also differed by sub-districts. Residents of Matlab South and Daudkandi were found to be more vulnerable to falls. This may be related to environmental factors. However, these were not captured in this survey, and this could be explored in future studies.

Results from the study may help in planning injury-prevention interventions and policies in Bangladesh. However, the findings of this study cannot be generalized to other areas in Bangladesh, as this study was conducted exclusively in rural Bangladesh. Previous studies have shown that rural areas have a higher burden of falls compared with urban areas [17,29]. Another limitation of the study could be the recall bias. In this study, the recall period for fatal and non-fatal fall was six and 12 months, respectively. Respondents are more likely to recall recent, severe, or fatal falls, and there may be underreporting. Other factors such as medication and substance use, or medical conditions such as poor vision, vertigo, stroke and musculoskeletal diseases, all may impair judgment, muscle strength, coordination or balance, and result in fall injuries [5]. Environmental factors such as poor infrastructure, building design, or lighting may also increase the risk of falling, especially for children who are inexperienced, and the elderly [5]. In this survey, data on these associated factors were not collected. While this study attempts to explore associations between fatal falls and sociodemographic factors, there may be some analytic limitations, as only 59 fatal falls were recorded in this survey.

5. Conclusions

Bangladesh has a high burden of fall-related mortality and morbidity. Populations at age extremes, and men in the productive age group, were found to be most vulnerable for falls. With increasing life expectancy, the burden of falls among the older population is expected to increase. Other groups that were vulnerable for falls included the widowed, those with lower education, unskilled/domestic laborers, students, and those in the lowest SES group. Interventions targeting these specific groups may help reduce the burden of falls in Bangladesh. Since most falls among children and elderly occur in the home environment, modifications in and around homes could be a potential strategy. Other strategies could be fall risk assessment and management. However, there is a dearth of evidence on the acceptability and effectiveness of these strategies in LMICs; as a result, future research on fall prevention interventions is suggested.

Acknowledgments: This work was conducted as part of the Saving of Lives from Drowning in Bangladesh study funded by the Bloomberg Philanthropies. The authors would like to thank our collaborators, Center for Injury Prevention and Research, Bangladesh and International Center for Diarrhoeal Disease Research, Bangladesh for their assistance with the study. We would also like to thank study participants.

Author Contributions: Shirin Wadhwaniya and Olakunle Alonge conceived this paper, contributed to data analysis and writing of the manuscript. Md. Kamran Ul Baset and Al-Amin Bhuiyan oversaw data collection and helped in revising the manuscript. Salim Chowdhury helped in developing and revising manuscript. Adnan A. Hyder contributed to data interpretation, helped in developing and revising manuscript, oversaw revisions and finalization. All authors provided editing support in finalizing the manuscript and have reviewed the final draft of the manuscript.

Conflicts of Interest: The authors declare no conflict of interest. The funding sponsors had no role in the design of the study; in the collection, analyses, or interpretation of data; in the writing of the manuscript, and in the decision to publish the results.

Abbreviations

aOR	Adjusted odds ratio
CIPRB	Center for Injury Prevention and Research, Bangladesh
CI	Confidence interval
icddr, b	International Center for Diarrhoeal Disease Research, Bangladesh
JHSPH	Johns Hopkins Bloomberg School of Public Health
LMIC	Low-and middle-income countries
MLR	Multivariate logistic regressions
OR	Odds ratio
SES	Socioeconomic status
YLD	Years lived with disability

References

1. GBD 2015 Mortality and Causes of Death Collaborators. Global, regional, and national life expectancy, all-cause mortality, and cause-specific mortality for 249 causes of death, 1980–2015: A systematic analysis for the Global Burden of Disease Study 2015. *Lancet* **2016**, *388*, 1459–1544.
2. Falls: Fact Sheet. Available online: http://www.who.int/mediacentre/factsheets/fs344/en/ (accessed on 18 April 2016).
3. Chandran, A.; Hyder, A.A.; Peek-Asa, C. The global burden of unintentional injuries and an agenda for progress. *Epidemiol. Rev.* **2010**, *32*, 110–120. [CrossRef] [PubMed]
4. *Injuries and Violence: The Facts 2014*; World Health Organization: Geneva, Switzerland, 2014. Available online: http://apps.who.int/iris/bitstream/10665/149798/1/9789241508018_eng.pdf (accessed on 22 July 2013).
5. *WHO Global Report on Falls Prevention in Older Age*; World Health Organization: Geneva, Switzerland, 2007. Available online: http://www.who.int/ageing/publications/Falls_prevention7March.pdf (accessed on 25 March 2014).

6. Hyder, A.A.; Sugerman, D.E.; Puvanachandra, P.; Razzak, J.; El-Sayed, H.; Isaza, A.; Rahman, F.; Peden, M. Global childhood unintentional injury surveillance in four cities in developing countries: A pilot study. *Bull. World Health Organ.* **2009**, *87*, 345–352. [CrossRef] [PubMed]

7. He, S.; Lunnen, J.C.; Puvanachandra, P.; Amar-Singh; Zia, N.; Hyder, A.A. Global childhood unintentional injury study: Multisite surveillance data. *Am. J. Public Health* **2014**, *103*, e79–84. [CrossRef] [PubMed]

8. Prevention of Injuries and Disabilities. Available online: http://www.searo.who.int/bangladesh/areas/injuriesanddisabilities/en/ (accessed on 10 September 2016).

9. Rahman, A.; Rahmna, A.F.; Shafinaz, S.; Linnan, M. Bangladesh Health and Injury Survey Report on Children. Available online: https://www.unicef.org/bangladesh/Bangladesh_Health_and_Injury_Survey-Report_on_Children.pdf (accessed on 27 April 2016).

10. Chowdhury, S.M.; Rahman, A.; Mashreky, S.R.; Giashuddin, S.M.; Svanstrm, L.; Hrte, L.G.; Rahman, F. The horizon of unintentional injuries among children in low-income setting: An overview from Bangladesh health and injury survey. *J. Environ. Public Health* **2009**. [CrossRef] [PubMed]

11. Rahman, F.; Andersson, R.; Svanström, L. Health impact of injuries: A population-based epidemiological investigation in a local community of Bangladesh. *J. Saf. Res.* **1998**, *29*, 213–222. [CrossRef]

12. Hyder, A.A.; Alonge, O.; He, S.; Wadhwaniya, S.; Rahman, F.; Rahman, A.; Arifeen, S.E. A framework for addressing implementation gap in global drowning prevention interventions: Experiences from Bangladesh. *J. Health Popul. Nutr.* **2014**, *32*, 564–576. [PubMed]

13. Hyder, A.A.; Alonge, O.; He, S.; Wadhwaniya, S.; Rahman, F.; Rahman, A.; Arifeen, S.E. Saving of children's lives from drowning project in Bangladesh. *Am. J. Prev. Med.* **2014**, *47*, 842–845. [CrossRef] [PubMed]

14. He, S.; Alonge, O.; Agrawal, P.; Sharmin, S.; Islam, I.; Mashreky, S.R.; Arifeen, S.E. Epidemiology of burns in rural Bangladesh: An update. *Int. J. Environ. Res. Public Health* **2017**, *14*, 381. [CrossRef] [PubMed]

15. Armitage, P.; Berry, G.; Mathhews, J.N.S. *Statistical Methods in Medical Research*, 4th ed.; Blackwell Science: Oxford, UK, 2002.

16. StataCorp. *Stata: Release 12*; StataCorp LP: College Station, TX, USA, 2011.

17. Chowdhury, S.M.; Rahman, A.; Mashreky, S.R.; Giashuddin, S.; Svanslröm, L.; Hörte, L.G.; Linnan, M.; Shafinaz, S.; Uhaa, I.J.; Rahman, A.K.M.F. Childhood fall: Epidemiologic findings from a population-based survey in Bangladesh. *Int. J. Disabil. Hum. Dev.* **2008**, *7*, 81–87. [CrossRef]

18. Chowdhury, S.M.; Svanström, L.; Hörte, L.G.; Chowdhury, R.A.; Rahman, F. Children's perceptions about falls and their prevention: A qualitative study from a rural setting in Bangladesh. *BMC Public Health* **2013**. [CrossRef] [PubMed]

19. World Bank Open Data. Available online: http://data.worldbank.org (accessed on 10 September 2016).

20. Jagnoor, J.; Keay, L.; Ivers, R. A slip and a trip? Falls in older people in Asia. *Injury* **2013**, *44*, 701–702. [CrossRef] [PubMed]

21. Chang, J.T.; Morton, S.C.; Rubenstein, L.Z.; Mojica, W.A.; Maglione, M.; Suttorp, M.J.; Roth, E.A.; Shekelle, P.G. Interventions for the prevention of falls in older adults: Systematic review and meta-analysis of randomised clinical trials. *BMJ* **2004**, *328*, 680. [CrossRef] [PubMed]

22. Jagnoor, J.; Keay, L.; Jaswal, N.; Kaur, M.; Ivers, R. A qualitative study on the perceptions of preventing falls as a health priority among older people in Northern India. *Inj. Prev.* **2014**, *20*, 29–34. [CrossRef] [PubMed]

23. Romli, M.H.; Tan, M.P.; Mackenzie, L.; Lovarini, M.; Suttanon, P.; Clemson, L. Falls amongst older people in Southeast Asia: A scoping review. *Public Health* **2017**, *145*, 96–112. [CrossRef] [PubMed]

24. Bachani, A.M.; Ghaffar, A.; Hyder, A.A. Burden of fall injuries in Pakistan—Analysis of the national injury survey of Pakistan. *East Mediterr. Health J.* **2011**, *17*, 375–381. [PubMed]

25. Pant, P.R.; Towner, E.; Pilkington, P.; Ellis, M. Epidemiology of unintentional child injuries in the South-East Asia Region: A systematic review. *Int. J. Inj. Control Saf. Promot.* **2015**, *22*, 24–32. [CrossRef] [PubMed]

26. Moshiro, C.; Heuch, I.; Åstrøm, A.N.; Setel, P.; Hemed, Y.; Kvåle, G. Injury morbidity in an urban and a rural area in Tanzania: An epidemiological survey. *BMC Public Health* **2005**. [CrossRef] [PubMed]

27. Fayyaz, J.; Wadhwaniya, S.; Shahzad, H.; Feroze, A.; Zia, N.; Mir, M.U.; Khan, U.R.; Iram, S.; Ali, S.; Razzak, J.A.; et al. Pattern of fall injuries in Pakistan: The Pakistan National Emergency Department Surveillance (Pak-NEDS) study. *BMC Emerg. Med.* **2015**. [CrossRef] [PubMed]

28. Shields, B.J.; Burkett, E.; Smith, G.A. Epidemiology of balcony fall-related injuries, United States, 1990–2006. *Am. J. Emerg. Med.* **2011**, *29*, 174–180. [CrossRef] [PubMed]
29. Stewart Williams, J.; Kowal, P.; Hestekin, H.; O'Driscoll, T.; Peltzer, K.; Yawson, A.; Biritwum, R.; Maximova, T.; Salinas Rodríguez, A.; Manrique Espinoza, B.; et al. Prevalence, risk factors and disability associated with fall-related injury in older adults in low-and middle-incomecountries: Results from the WHO Study on global AGEing and adult health (SAGE). *BMC Med.* **2015**. [CrossRef] [PubMed]

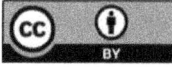

International Journal of
Environmental Research and Public Health

MDPI

Article

The Burden of Suicide in Rural Bangladesh: Magnitude and Risk Factors

Shumona Sharmin Salam [1,*], Olakunle Alonge [2], Md Irteja Islam [1], Dewan Md Emdadul Hoque [1], Shirin Wadhwaniya [2], Md Kamran Ul Baset [3], Saidur Rahman Mashreky [3] and Shams El Arifeen [1]

[1]   International Centre for Diarrhoeal Disease Research, GPO Box 128, Dhaka 1000, Bangladesh; irteja.islam@icddrb.org (M.I.I.); emdad@icddrb.org (D.M.E.H.); shams@icddrb.org (S.E.A.)
[2]   Department of International Health, Johns Hopkins University Bloomberg School of Public Health, Baltimore, MA 21205, USA; oalonge1@jhu.edu (O.A.); swadhwa2@jhu.edu (S.W.)
[3]   Center for Injury Prevention and Research, House # B-162, Road # 23, New DOHS, Mohakhali, Dhaka 1206, Bangladesh; kamran_baset@yahoo.co.uk (M.K.U.B.); mashreky@ciprb.org (S.R.M.)
*   Correspondence: shumona@icddrb.org

Received: 5 July 2017; Accepted: 6 September 2017; Published: 9 September 2017

Abstract: The aim of the paper is to quantify the burden and risk factors of fatal and non-fatal suicidal behaviors in rural Bangladesh. A census was carried out in seven sub-districts encompassing 1.16 million people. Face-to-face interviews were conducted at the household level. Descriptive analyses were done to quantify the burden and Poisson regression was run to determine on risk factors. The estimated rates of fatal and non-fatal suicide were 3.29 and 9.86 per 100,000 person years (PY) observed, respectively. The risk of suicide was significantly higher by 6.31 times among 15–17 and 4.04 times among 18–24 olds compared to 25–64 years old. Married adolescents were 22 times more likely to commit suicide compared to never-married people. Compared to Chandpur/Comilla district, the risk of suicide was significantly higher in Narshingdi. Students had significantly lower risk of non-fatal suicidal behavior compared to skilled laborers. The risk of non-fatal suicidal behavior was lower in Sherpur compared to Chandpur/Comilla. Among adolescents, unskilled laborers were 16 times more likely to attempt suicide than students. The common methods for fatal and non-fatal suicidal behaviors were hanging and poisoning. Suicide is a major public health problem in Bangladesh that needs to be addressed with targeted interventions.

Keywords: suicide; attempted suicide; burden; risk factors; rural; Bangladesh; injury; violence

---

1. Introduction

According to the 2014 WHO Global Health Estimates, there were about 803,900 suicides in 2012 representing 1.4% of the global burden of disease or over 39 million disability adjusted life years (DALYs) lost [1]. Fatal suicidal behavior or suicide is death resulting from self-harm. Worldwide, suicide accounted for 16% of injury mortality and 1.4% of total mortality in 2012, making it the 15th most common cause of death for all age groups in that year [1,2]. Analysis of trends indicate that the overall suicide rate has decreased significantly over the past decade. The global suicide rate was 11.4 per 100,000 population in 2012, a decrease from 14.4 per 100,000 in 2000 [1]. However, the rate of decline flat-lined in the latter part of that decade, and the rate in 2008 (11.6 per 100,000) was about the same as rate reported for 2012 [3–5]. Globally, suicide remains the second leading cause of death among 15–29 year olds [1,2]. In addition to these striking facts for suicide, there are indications that, for every adult that dies by suicide, there are 10–20 more who attempted a suicide event [2,5]. This assumption for suicide attempts is based on the WHO world mental health surveys among adults (>18 years of age) in 21 low-middle and high-income countries who report a prevalence of 3–4 per 1000 individuals [6].

Fatal and non-fatal suicidal behaviors have been found be mostly prevalent among the vulnerable populations of the world where availability of and accessibility to resources and services for identification and treatment are scarce [2]. In fact, three-fourths of the global suicides have been estimated to occur in low and middle-income countries (LMICs) [2]. The southeast Asia region alone accounts for 40% of the global suicide deaths, with China and India being the leading contributors [2,4]. Although there are variations in trends and risk factors of suicide among countries in the southeast Asia region, compared to Western countries, the region as whole has higher suicide rates, lower gender (male-to-female) suicide rate gap, higher rates among the elderly, and an increasing trend of youth suicides [5,7]. Reviews and epidemiological data also indicate that there exists wide urban-rural disparity in suicide, with suicide rates often greater in rural areas [5,8,9].

Like most southeast Asian countries, a fundamental challenge for Bangladesh is the lack of quality suicide data or system for monitoring and surveillance. In Bangladesh, a limited number of studies have attempted to quantify suicide rates. Mashreky et al. suggested that about 10,000 people commit suicide in the country in a year [10], and the rate of suicide was found to be 7.3 per 100,000 population (6.5 in males and 8.2 in females) and was highest in the 60+ age group and considerably high among adolescents [10]. These estimates for were based on the 2003 Bangladesh Health and Injury Survey [10]. According to WHO Global Health Estimates, the suicide rate for 2012 in Bangladesh was 7.8 per 100,000 population (8.7 in females and 6.8 in males) [11]. Demographic and health surveillance in two rural sub-districts of Bangladesh between 2004 and 2010 revealed that the most common cause of death for young adults (aged 15–49) was injury (23.5%) with suicide accounting for 11.9% [12]. Other studies that have attempted to determine the causes of female deaths, revealed a growing rate of suicide among adolescent females [13]. Analysis of results from national household surveys in 2001 and 2010 and hospital based surveys in 1996–1997 suggested that suicide was the main cause for deaths among adolescent females, accounting for 16–22% of all deaths in this age group [13]. There is a need for recent population-based data that could be used to define the burden and epidemiology of suicide in Bangladesh, and to consequently address interventions for reducing rates of fatal and non-fatal suicidal behavior in Bangladesh.

The objective of this paper is to quantify the burden and socio-demographic risk factors of fatal and non-fatal suicidal behaviors in rural Bangladesh. The goal is to identify high-risk subgroups, demonstrate any transition in causes of death in the country and to call for action on the need to recognize and address this enormous public health issue on a national scale. It is hoped that this paper will provide evidence to influence national policies to address and invest in related research and preventive approaches.

2. Materials and Methods

2.1. Study Design, Area and Population

The data for this paper is from an implementation research study conducted with an aim to reduce drowning in under-five children in five districts of rural Bangladesh [14,15]. A cross-sectional baseline census was conducted over a six months period from June through November 2013 before the start of the implementation of the drowning prevention interventions [16]. The census covered 1.165 million people in 51 unions from seven sub-districts of Bangladesh (and this study describing the epidemiology of fatal and nonfatal suicide behaviors is based on the census). The sub-districts included were Matlab North, Matlab South, Daudkandi, Chandpur Sadar, and Manohardi in the central section of the country, and Raiganj and Sherpur in the north.

2.2. Questionnaire and Data Collection

The baseline census collected information on fatal and non-fatal injury outcomes including fatal and non-fatal suicidal behaviors, characteristics of the underlying injury mechanisms and health seeking behavior for the injury or death outcome on all populations in the census area. In addition, the census collected information on social and demographic characteristics, physical environment and birth history. This was done using a questionnaire covering seven modules (I. Household characteristics and socioeconomic census; II. Birth history; III. Household environment, IV. Death confirmation; V. Injury morbidity; VI. Injury mortality and VII. Injury mechanisms). The injury mechanisms module (module VII) comprised of 12 forms covering 12 injury events, the first of which was attempted suicide. In addition, there were three notification forms: injury notification, death notification and child notification, which provided notifications of any injuries or deaths including suicide and attempted suicide from module I. All fatal injury information (including fatal suicidal behavior) was collected over a one-year recall period, whereas non-fatal injuries (including non-fatal suicidal behavior) were collected over a six-month recall period.

Suicide (or non-fatal suicidal behavior) was operationally defined as a self-initiated injury event that resulted in a fatal outcome (or non-fatal outcome). The injury events assessed were defined based on ICD-10 classification, and are described in details elsewhere [16].

All information was collected directly from the head of households or any adults 18 years above with sufficient knowledge of the household. All forms were written in English and translated to Bangla. The forms were back-translated and pilot-tested prior to the actual data collection.

Data collection was implemented by two sets of trained data collectors. The first set of data collectors completed the questionnaire forms in module I–III and notified of any fatal suicide or non-fatal suicide events. In module I after enlisting all the household members and their soico-demographic information, we asked "whether the member had suffered from any non-fatal injuries (read out all injuries) in the past six months". In order to obtain information on deaths we asked "whether there were any deaths in the past one year". Based on the notification, a second set of data collectors completed the questionnaire forms in module IV–VII only in households with the suicide injury or death event. Each set of the questionnaire forms took between 40–50 min to complete. Written informed consent was obtained prior to data collection.

2.3. Statistical Method and Analyses

Descriptive statistics were used to describe the population by various variables such as age, gender, marital status, educational attainment, wealth quintile and geographical area. The overall rates of suicide and attempted suicide was calculated per 100,000 person years observed (PYO). The mortality and morbidity rates were also stratified by the above-mentioned variables. Principal component analysis was done to estimate the wealth quintile using various variables that indicate asset availability and housing conditions.

Multivariable analysis was performed with multilevel Poisson regression models. Model estimates were reported as incidence rate ratios (IRR), with their respective 95% confidence intervals. The models were first implemented with one covariate, and then adjusted for other covariates and possible confounders (age, gender, marital status, educational attainment, wealth quintile and geographical area). Age, education and occupation were considered as categorical variables, whereas gender was considered as a binary predictor (male as reference group). Socioeconomic quintile was considered as ordinal data from lowest to highest. Age was theorized to modify the risk of fatal and non-fatal suicidal behavior with regards to other variables, especially marital status in rural Bangladesh. Thus, separate analyses were implemented for (1) individuals 15 years and older, and (2) adolescents-only (aged 10–17 years) to adjust for the possible interactions with age. The final results for individuals above 15 years of age are presented in the paper, and results for the adolescent-only analyses have been included in the (Supplementary Materials Tables S1 and S2).

Variable construction and estimations were done with the statistical software STATA 13 (Stata Corp. 2013. Stata Statistical Software: Release 13. College Station, TX, USA: Stata Corp LP.).

2.4. Ethical Statement

Ethical approval was obtained from of the Institutional Review Board of the Johns Hopkins Bloomberg School of Public Health (JHSPH) (ethics approval code is 00004746); and Ethics Review Committees of International Centre for Diarrhoeal Disease Research, Bangladesh (icddr,b) and Center for Injury Prevention and Research Bangladesh (CIPRB) under the study Saving of Lives from Drowning (SoLiD), Bangladesh.

3. Results

The survey covered a population of 1,169,593 (Table 1). Overall, 21.6% of the population was less than 10 years of age, 72.3% were between 10–65 years of age and only 6.1% of the population was above 65 years. More than three-fifth (65%) of the respondents had received at least primary education and about half (48.8%) of the population were married during the time of the survey. Three-fourths (74.6%) of the population were not employed and were either retired, unemployed, housewives, students or children. Among those who were employed, a majority were involved in agricultural activities (9%), followed by skilled work (7.6%) and business (5.3%). Household wealth quintiles were evenly distributed. The majority of respondents resided in Matlab North (22.7), Sherpur (19.5%), Matlab South (17.9%) and Manohardi (17.5%) sub-districts of the country.

Table 1. Socio-demographic characteristics of the respondents.

Characteristics	N = 1,169,593	%
Age (in years)		
<10	252,392	21.6
10–14	142,121	12.2
15–17	62,098	5.3
18–24	133,534	11.4
25–64	508,059	43.4
65+	71,389	6.1
Sex		
Male	567,674	48.5
Female	601,919	51.5
Education [1]		
No education	295,314	25.3
Primary complete (five years)	407,923	34.9
Secondary complete (10 years)	289,658	24.8
Secondary and above	63,873	5.5
Under five children	112,664	9.6
Occupation [2]		
Agriculture	104,956	9.0
Business	61,661	5.3
Skilled labor	89,151	7.6
Unskilled labor	24,520	2.1
Transport worker	17,037	1.5
Students	312,537	26.7
Retired/unemployed/housewife	408,583	35.0
Children	144,454	12.4
Others (NA)	5948	0.5
Marital Status		
Married (Reference)	571,206	48.8
Never-married	227,319	19.4
Widowed/Divorced/Separated	59,033	5.0
Children (<12 years)	312,035	26.7

Table 1. *Cont.*

Characteristics	N = 1,169,593	%
Wealth quintile		
Lowest	211,601	18.1
Second	218,695	18.7
Middle	238,371	20.4
Fourth	247,716	21.2
Highest	253,210	21.6
Sub-district		
Matlab North	265,897	22.7
Matlab South	209,772	17.9
Chandpur Sadar	128,356	11.0
Raiganj	104,357	8.9
Sherpur	228,519	19.5
Manohardi	204,319	17.5
Daudkandi	28,373	2.4
District		
Chandpur/Comilla	632,398	54.1
Sirajganj	104,357	8.9
Sherpur	228,519	19.5
Narshingdi	204,319	17.5

[1] Information on education missing for 0.01 (161) participants; [2] Information on occupation missing for 0.06 (746) participants.

A total of 38 fatal suicide and 57 non-fatal suicidal events were recorded in the past one year and six months prior to the survey, respectively (Table 2). In rural Bangladesh, the estimated rates of fatal and non-fatal suicidal behavior were 3.29 per 100,000 PYO and 9.86 per 100,000 PYO. Suicide rates were found to be higher among the younger population specifically the adolescents compared to the adults and the elderly. The rates were highest among 15–17 year olds (11.3 per 100,000 PYO), followed by 18–24 year olds (7.5 per 100,000 PYO) and 3.52 per 100,000 PYO among young adolescents (aged between 10–14 years old). There was no difference in the rates of fatal suicidal behavior comparing males and females of all ages, and the gender ratio (male-to-female) was 1.18. The rates did not vary much by marital status and no definitive pattern in suicidal behavior was observed by education or wealth quintile. The rate was highest among those who had completed 10 years of education or had no education, and among those belonging to the middle wealth quintile. The suicide rate was found to be high among the transport workers (17.66 per 100,000 PYO), but was similar among other occupations, ranging from 3.38 in skilled labors to 4.80 in those involved in agricultural activities. Geographically, suicide rates were found to be higher in Raiganj and Manohardi Sub-districts in Northern Bangladesh compared to the sub-districts of Matlab situated in central Bangladesh.

Table 2. Distribution of suicide and attempted suicide rates by socio-demographic and geographical factors, rural Bangladesh.

Characteristics	N	Fatal Suicidal Behavior			Non-Fatal Suicidal Behavior		
		Person Years Observed (PYO)	Frequency	Mortality Rate per 100,000 Person Years Observed (PYO)	Person Years Observed (PYO)	Frequency	Morbidity Rate per 100,000 Person Years Observed (PYO)
Total	1,169,593	1,153,901	38	3.29	578,046	57	9.86
Age (in years)							
<10	252,392	240,739	0	0.00	122,966	0	0.00
10–14	142,121	141,849	5	3.52	70,894	4	5.64
15–17	62,098	61,972	7	11.30	30,965	4	12.92
18–24	133,534	133,247	10	7.50	66,568	13	19.53
25–64	508,059	506,348	14	2.76	252,581	34	13.46
65+	71,389	69,745	2	2.87	34,072	2	5.87
Sex							
Male	567,674	559,566	20	3.57	280,538	28	9.98
Female	601,919	594,335	18	3.03	297,508	29	9.75
Education [1]							
No education	295,314	293,176	11	3.75	145,672	16	10.98
Primary complete (five years)	407,923	406,727	9	2.21	203,011	17	8.37
Secondary complete (10 years)	289,658	288,858	17	5.89	144,209	22	15.26
Secondary and above	63,873	63,690	1	1.57	31,787	2	6.29
Under five children	112,664	101,294	0	0.00	53,291	0	0.00
Occupation [2]							
Agriculture	104,956	104,221	5	4.80	51,802	11	21.23
Business	61,661	61,397	0	0.00	30,600	1	3.27
Skilled labor	89,151	88,864	3	3.38	44,330	8	18.05
Unskilled labor	24,520	24,417	1	4.10	12,169	4	32.87
Transport worker	17,037	16,989	3	17.66	8480	1	11.79
Students	312,537	311,935	12	3.85	155,892	6	3.85
Retired/Unemployed/Housewife	408,583	406,478	14	3.44	202,394	26	12.85
Children (Under 12 years)	144,454	133,003	0	0.00	69,125	0	0.00
Others (NA)	5948	5857	0	0.00	2886	0	0.00

Table 2. *Cont.*

Characteristics	N	Fatal Suicidal Behavior			Non-Fatal Suicidal Behavior		
		Person Years Observed (PYO)	Frequency	Mortality Rate per 100,000 Person Years Observed (PYO)	Person Years Observed (PYO)	Frequency	Morbidity Rate per 100,000 Person Years Observed (PYO)
Marital Status							
Married	571,206	568,601	25	4.40	283,292	37	13.06
Never-married	227,319	226,802	11	4.85	113,320	15	13.24
Widowed/Divorced/Separated	59,033	58,192	0	0.00	28,705	3	10.45
Children (Under 12 years)	312,035	300,306	2	0.67	152,729	2	1.31
Wealth quintile							
Lowest	211,601	208,601	7	3.36	104,479	10	9.57
Second	218,695	215,949	5	2.32	108,190	13	12.02
Middle	238,371	235,239	10	4.25	117,830	14	11.88
Fourth	247,716	244,482	9	3.68	122,460	11	8.98
Highest	253,210	249,630	7	2.80	125,088	9	7.19
Sub-district							
Matlab North	265,897	262,510	7	2.67	131,406	11	8.37
Matlab South	209,772	206,600	5	2.42	103,492	14	13.53
Chandpur Sadar	128,356	126,659	3	2.37	63,475	5	7.88
Raiganj	104,357	103,052	5	4.85	51,612	11	21.31
Sherpur	228,519	225,476	6	2.66	113,055	4	3.54
Manohardi	204,319	201,641	12	5.95	101,004	12	11.88
Daudkandi	28,373	27,962	0	0.00	14,002	0	0.00
District							
Chandpur/Comilla	632,398	623,732	15	2.40	312,375	30	9.60
Sirajganj	104,357	103,052	5	4.85	51,612	11	21.31
Sherpur	228,519	225,476	6	2.66	113,055	4	3.54
Narshingdi	204,319	201,641	12	5.95	101,004	12	11.88

[1] Information on education missing for 0.01 (161) participants; [2] Information on occupation missing for 0.06 (746) participants.

Table 3 presents stratified analysis of suicide rates by age and sex. Among males, suicide rates are highest among the 15–17 year olds followed by 10–14 year olds, whereas among females the rates are highest among the 15–17 year olds and 18–24 year olds. The rates of suicide are higher in females among 15–24 year olds than in males of the same age group. The rates are, however, higher in males for 10–14 and 25–64 year olds.

Table 3. Suicide rates by age and sex, rural Bangladesh.

Age Group (Years)	Male				Female			
	PYO	Suicide (*n*)	Mortality Rate/100,000 PYO	Confidence Interval (CI)	PYO	Suicide (*n*)	Mortality Rate/100,000 PYO	Confidence Interval (CI)
<10	122,970	0	0.00		117,769	0	0.00	
10–14	72,339	4	5.53	1.51–14.16	69,510	1	1.44	0.04–8.02
15–17	33,156	3	9.05	1.87–26.44	28,815	4	13.88	3.78–35.54
18–24	57,909	3	5.18	1.07–15.14	75,339	7	9.29	3.74–19.14
25–64	236,636	9	3.80	1.74–7.22	269,712	5	1.85	0.60–4.33
65+	36,556	1	2.74	0.07–15.24	33,189	1	3.01	0.08–16.79
Total	559,566	20	3.57	2.18–5.52	594,335	18	3.03	1.79–4.79

In contrast to suicide rates, the rates of non-fatal suicidal behavior were highest among individuals aged 18–24 year olds (19.53 per 100,000 PYO), 25–64 year olds (13.46 per 100,000 PYO) followed by 15–17 year olds (12.92 per 100,000 PYO). The rates were highest in people involved in un-skilled labor (32.87 per 100,000 PYO) and agricultural activities (21.23 per 100,000 PYO) and more common in people belonging to the bottom three wealth quintiles. Non-fatal suicidal behavior was also evident among women who were widowed, divorced or separated (10.45 per 100,000 PYO), which was not present in the case of suicide. Along with Raiganj (21.31 per 100,000 PYO) and Manohardi (11.88 per 100,000 PYO) sub-districts, the rates were also high in Matlab South (13.53 per 100,000 PYO).

Table 4 presents crude and adjusted IRR for fatal suicide and non-fatal suicidal behavior among respondents aged 15 years or more in the study. The significant factors associated with fatal suicidal behavior in the adjusted model included age, and geographical region (Table 4). The adjusted risk of fatal suicidal behavior was clearly higher, by six and four times among the 15–17 year olds (IRR 6.31, CI 1.35–29.32) and 18–24 year olds (IRR 4.04, CI 1.56–10.47) respectively, compared to those aged between 25–64 years old. In addition, the risk was significantly higher in the Narshingdi district (IRR 2.89, CI 1.26–6.65) compared to Chandpur/Comilla district. Although transport workers were more likely to commit suicide compared to skilled labor, the relationship was not significant in the adjusted model. In addition, adjusted analysis only among adolescents aged between 10–17 year olds revealed that the risk of fatal suicidal behavior was 22 times higher among those who were married compared to those who were never-married (IRR 22.06, CI 3.70–131.63) (Supplementary Materials Table S1).

Table 4. Unadjusted and adjusted analysis for fatal suicidal behavior by socio-demographic and geographical factors, rural Bangladesh.

Characteristics	Unadjusted		Adjusted	
	Incidence Rate Ratio (IRR)	95% CI	Incidence Rate Ratio (IRR)	95% CI
Age (in years)				
15–17	4.09 **	1.64–10.12	6.31 *	1.35–29.32
18–24	2.71 *	1.2–6.11	4.04 *	1.56–10.47
25–64	Reference		Reference	
65+	1.04	0.24–4.56	1.48	0.32–6.87

Table 4. *Cont.*

Characteristics	Unadjusted		Adjusted	
	Incidence Rate Ratio (IRR)	95% CI	Incidence Rate Ratio (IRR)	95% CI
Sex				
Male	1.05	0.53–2.08	0.87	0.29–2.56
Female	Reference		Reference	
Education				
No education	2.81	0.36–21.75	5.48	0.56–53.10
Primary complete (five years)	1.50	0.17–12.83	2.27	0.22–22.62
Secondary complete (10 years)	4.15	0.54–31.25	4.04	0.49–32.97
Secondary and above	Reference		Reference	
Occupation				
Agriculture	1.40	0.33–5.84	0.99	0.22–4.45
Business	0.00		0.00	
Skilled labor	Reference		Reference	
Unskilled labor	1.25	0.13–12.01	1.20	0.12–11.82
Transport worker	5.14 *	1.03–25.48	4.25	0.82–21.82
Students	2.89	0.76–10.88	1.86	0.32–10.67
Retired/Unemployed/Housewife	0.95	0.27–3.33	0.62	0.13–2.87
Children (Under 12 years)	0.00		0.00	
Others (NA)	0.00		0.00	
Marital Status				
Married	0.68	0.31–1.47	3.60	0.92–14.06
Never-married	Reference		Reference	
Widowed/Divorced/Separated	0.00		0.00	
Wealth quintile				
Lowest	Reference		Reference	
Second	0.76	0.20–2.83	0.76	0.20–2.85
Middle	1.55	0.52–4.61	1.71	0.55–5.26
Fourth	1.44	0.48–4.28	1.61	0.51–5.07
Highest	0.92	0.28–3.01	1.03	0.28–3.71
District				
Chandpur/Comilla	Reference		Reference	
Sirajganj	2.48	0.87–7.02	2.32	0.77–6.88
Sherpur	1.19	0.41–3.37	0.97	0.33–2.89
Narshingdi	2.83 *	1.24–6.42	2.89 *	1.26–6.65

* $p < 0.05$; ** $p < 0.01$.

The two factors that were significantly associated with non-fatal suicidal behavior in both the adjusted model among respondents aged 15 years or older included occupation and districts (Table 5). Compared to those involved in skilled labor, students were found to have a significantly lower risk (adjusted) of non-fatal suicidal behavior (IRR 0.21, CI 0.04–1.00). People living in Sherpur were found to be at significantly lower risk compared to those living in Chandpur/Comilla sub-districts (IRR 0.28, CI 0.08–0.94). Although, the risk of non-fatal suicidal behavior was twice among people living in Sirajganj district compared to those living in Chandpur/Comilla districts (IRR 2.10, CI 1.01–4.36) in the unadjusted model, the relationship was not significant in the adjusted model. Among adolescents aged 10–17 years, the risk of non-fatal suicidal behavior (adjusted) was 16 times higher among those involved in unskilled labor compared to students (IRR 15.75. CI 1.35–184.52) (Supplementary Materials Table S2).

Table 5. Unadjusted and adjusted analysis of non-fatal suicidal behavior by socio-demographic and geographical factors, rural Bangladesh.

Characteristics	Unadjusted		Adjusted	
	Incidence Rate Ratio (IRR)	95% CI	Incidence Rate Ratio (IRR)	95% CI
Age (in years)				
15–17	0.97	0.34–2.72	1.01	0.25–4.03
18–24	1.46	0.77–2.77	1.31	0.59–2.91
25–64	Reference		Reference	
65+	0.44	0.10–0.82	0.49	0.11–2.18
Sex				
Male	1.07	0.63–1.84	0.63	0.24–1.67
Female	Reference		Reference	
Education				
No education	1.91	0.44–8.35	1.59	0.31–8.02
Primary complete (5 years)	2.23	0.51–9.75	1.60	0.45–2.00
Secondary complete (10 years)	2.71	0.64–11.55	2.28	0.66–3.03
Secondary and above	Reference			
Occupation				
Agriculture	1.15	0.46–2.87	1.49	0.56–3.97
Business	0.18	0.02–1.43	0.20	0.03–1.69
Skilled labor	Reference		Reference	
Unskilled labor	1.87	0.56–6.21	2.25	0.66–7.68
Transport worker	0.63	0.08–5.10	0.78	0.10–6.38
Students	0.41	0.10–1.54	0.21 *	0.04–1.00
Retired/Unemployed/Housewife	0.69	0.31–1.53	0.57	0.19–1.72
Children (Under 12 years)	0.00		0.00	
Others (NA)	0.00		0.00	
Marital Status				
Married	0.72	0.39–1.37	0.55	0.22–1.38
Never-married	Reference		Reference	
Widowed/Divorced/Separated	0.58	0.17–2.04	0.6	0.13–2.86
Children < 12 years	0.00			
Wealth quintile				
Lowest	Reference		Reference	
Second	1.27	0.53–3.00	1.17	0.49–2.80
Middle	1.15	0.48–2.71	1.12	0.46–2.71
Fourth	0.98	0.40–2.35	0.99	0.40–2.45
Highest	0.77	0.30–1.94	0.82	0.30–2.19
District				
Chandpur/Comilla	Reference		Reference	
Sirajganj	2.11 *	1.02–4.34	2.06	0.96–4.42
Sherpur	0.31	0.09–1.01	0.28 *	0.08–0.94
Narshingdi	1.34	0.68–2.63	1.34	0.67–2.66

* $p < 0.05$; ** $p < 0.01$.

The most common method of suicide was hanging (59%) followed by poisoning (31%), burn (5.1%), drowning (2.6%) and exsanguination (2.6%). These frequencies were reversed for non-fatal suicidal behavior, where poisoning (71.93%) was the most common method followed by hanging (22.81%), implying that the survival rate was higher among those who attempted to use poisoning as the method. Pesticides were the most commonly used poisoning material (62.7% in case of non-fatal suicidal behavior and 83% in case of fatal suicidal behavior). About two-thirds of the cases undertook the events at home followed by in-laws and other's house (about one-fifth) and only a small proportion of cases chose public places for the event. There were no differences in the methods and place by gender and the pattern was similar.

4. Discussion

This paper set out to explore the epidemiology of fatal and non-fatal suicidal behavior in rural Bangladesh. The estimated rates of fatal and non-fatal suicidal behavior were 3.29 and 9.86 per 100,000 PYO, respectively. The significant factors associated with fatal suicidal behavior included age, marital status and geographical region, whereas the two factors that were significantly associated with non-fatal suicidal behavior were occupation and districts.

The estimated rate for fatal suicidal behavior was 3.29 per 100,000 PYO (3.25 per 100,000 population per year), whereas the rate for non-fatal suicidal behavior was 9.86 per 100,000 PYO (4.87 per 100,000 population per six months) indicating that approximately 5000 people lost their lives to suicide and another 15,000 attempted a non-fatal suicide event in 2013. This rate for fatal suicidal behavior was, however, two times lower than the overall rate presented in the Global Health Estimates for 2012 [1] and almost four times lower than the rate of suicide in rural Bangladesh reported by Mashreky et al. [10]. Perhaps, this may be because the current data is only representative of rural Bangladesh, and significant differences may exist in suicide rates between urban and rural populations in Bangladesh. In addition, the rates are lower than that of other Asian countries such as China (9.8) [8], India (22.0) [9], South Korea (31.0), Japan (24.0), Sri Lanka (23.0), Taiwan (17.6), and Hong Kong (13.8) [5,8]. The rural rates in several of these Asian countries, including China, India, Sri Lanka, Japan, and Taiwan have been found to be higher compared to urban rates [5,8,9]. Disaggregation by gender and age reveals further disparity in urban-rural rates in these countries. Several contextual factors have been described to contribute to the increased risk of suicide in rural areas, including socio-economic and cultural differences, availability and accessibility to services, access to means, and, community attitudes towards mental illness and care-seeking [17–19] The rates presented for different countries should be interpreted with caution since only a few countries in the world have good vital registration or data collection systems that help obtain high quality data. For example, estimates in countries such as Hong Kong, Japan, Malaysia, Singapore, South Korea, and Taiwan are considered to be more reliable compared to countries such as China, India, Thailand and Sri Lanka [5]. The situation is further complicated by issues such as stigmatization and illegality that result in misclassification and under-reporting of suicide and suicidal attempts. It must be noted that Bangladesh is predominantly a Muslim country with not only strong religious sanctions against suicide and suicidal attempts but also has punitive laws against attempted suicide (Bangladesh penal code, 1860).

The gender gap (male to female ratio) for suicide was very low at 1.2. The findings contrast with High Income Countries (HIC), where suicide rates for males are about 3–4 times higher than those for females but similar to other Low and Middle Income Countries (LMICs) where the gender gap is low (1.6) [2,4,20,21]. Several Asian countries such as China, Hong Kong, Japan, India, Taiwan, Singapore, and Sri Lanka also have a lower gender ratio although there is some evidence that the gap may be increasing [5,7,8,22,23]. There are many potential reasons for different suicide rates in men and women: gender equality issues, differences in socially acceptable methods of dealing with stress and conflict for men and women, availability of and preference for different means of suicide, availability and patterns of alcohol consumption, and differences in care-seeking rates for mental disorders between men and women.

Our study also revealed that risks of fatal and non-fatal suicidal behavior were higher among the young, including the adolescents especially those 15–17 year olds, and young adults 18–24 year olds. The rates of suicide varied by age and sex with female 15–24 year olds individuals to be more likely to commit suicide compared to their male counterparts. Several studies in Bangladesh have also attempted to highlight this issue indicating that the young people, and not the elderly, are particularly vulnerable to injuries including self-harm and suicide in the country [12,13,24–27]. Despite this, there has been no study in Bangladesh that has aimed to determine the factors influencing high suicide rates among adolescents and young adults.

We conducted separate regression analysis among adolescents age 10–17 years and found early marriage to significant stressor for suicide, which explains why the suicide burden affect the female adolescents more. Such high suicide rates among adolescent women may be because of early and forced marriage, marital abuse related to dowry, and complete lack of opportunity for advancement and development coupled with the tendency to impulsive behavior and actions that is typical of young adolescents. Several studies, particularly in the West and developed regions, indicate that marriage is protective [28–31], while others in many developing countries indicate that it is a significant source of abuse and stress, particularly for the women, leading to higher psychiatric morbidity, suicidal ideation and suicide [9,32–39]. Our study did not find marriage to be protective of suicide for women of all ages. In addition, we found non-fatal suicidal behavior rates to be higher in adolescents who were involved in unskilled labor compared to those who were students. Psychological, familial, social, and cultural factors risk factors that have been identified to influence adolescents to commit suicide include low socio-economic and educational status, family history of suicide, parental separation, divorce, or death, poor relationship with family and peers, social contagion, prevalence of psychiatric disorder, psychological stressors, sexual abuse, substance abuse, social deprivation, and availability of high lethality methods (e.g., guns) [27,40–42]. Another emerging issue is the media representation of suicidal behavior including the modern internet that have been found to have substantial influence on the vulnerable including adolescents in some Asian countries [40,43].

Although not significant, the rates of fatal and non-fatal suicidal behavior were very high among agricultural workers and unskilled labor. Compared to skilled laborers students were, however, found to have lower rates of non-fatal suicidal behavior. This needs further attention and research since several studies have indicated that acute life stressors and poor educational status are significantly associated with higher rates of fatal and non-fatal suicidal behavior [5,21,44,45]. A variation was also seen geographically where fatal and non-fatal suicidal rates were found to be more in Sirajganj and Narsingdi districts of the country indicating the need to provide attention to particular socio-demographic or other factors in the regions.

Studies reporting methods of suicide indicate that availability of and accessibility to methods influence the choice of the method and act as factor in increasing overall fatal and non-fatal suicidal events [46]. As such, the common suicide methods not only vary by age and sex but also shift with the availability/restriction of new methods and technologies [47]. Globally, ingestion of pesticide, hanging and firearms are among the most common methods of suicide, whereas poisoning and hanging has been found to be most common in Asia [2,5,7,47,48]. Our study findings are consistent with those in Asia and reports hanging followed by poisoning to be the most common methods for suicide. For non-fatal suicidal behavior, the most common method was poisoning followed by hanging. Rural economy in Bangladesh is predominantly agricultural where availability of pesticides is rampant and unregulated. Several studies have indicated that, despite some challenges, means restriction through legal regulations, safe storage, awareness could be an important strategy for controlling fatal and non-fatal suicidal behavior at the population level [43,46,49,50]. For example, restrictions on the import and sales of pesticides in Sri Lanka resulted in reductions in suicide in both men and women of all ages with 19,769 fewer suicides occurring in 1996–2005 compared to 1986–1995 [51]. In addition to this research on suicide prevention also indicates the need for national strategy and community based approaches focusing on targeted groups [52,53]. The application of findings of prevention studies from other countries should be interpreted with caution given the unique sociocultural context of Bangladesh, and implementation research on suicide prevention in the country is required.

Limitations and Challenges

The study was conducted in rural Bangladesh and might not be generalizable for the country as risk factors might be very different in urban Bangladesh. Our study findings are generalizable to rural

Bangladesh and similar settings in other low and middle income countries The fatal and non-fatal suicide rates, especially for non-fatal suicidal behavior, may be underreported due to challenges in data collection, recall bias, stigmatization and for punitive reasons. Given that information obtained from the head of the households may be subject to recall and social desirability biases, and to avoid stigma and likely legal punishments, suicide (especially of children and adolescent females) may be underreported, leading to biased fatal and nonfatal suicide rates. Contemporaneous and real-time death review/social autopsy may provide less biased estimates. Although mental illness is widely accepted as a risk factor of fatal and non-fatal suicidal behavior, our study was not designed to elicit any information on mental illness.

5. Conclusions

This study has made an attempt to provide updated information on the burden of suicide and suicidal attempts from a population census that covered almost 1.2 million rural people in five districts of the country. We conclude that suicide is a serious public health problem in Bangladesh especially among the high-risk individuals such as adolescent women and married women; some of the factors associated with completed and attempted suicide are similar or vary compared to other Asian and LMIC countries. Considering the context, where resources and services for suicide identification, treatment and support are limited, there is a need to develop targeted national strategies and action plans, prevention programs and conduct further research to learn more about the constraints and reduce the rate of suicide and its associated risk factors. Strategies to uplift the status of women in rural Bangladesh, such as creating opportunities that would improve financial independence, programs to create awareness of mental health issues and access to mental health treatment among married adolescent women, are among a few potential paths to take to address the huge public health burden of suicide. Further research to adequately characterize the burden of suicide and the gender disparities in suicide and attempted suicide rates in the country are needed. Implementation research on community-based prevention strategies, such as counseling/support groups and mental health awareness, is also needed to support the development of a national strategy.

There is also an urgent need to establish reliable systems to continuously collect data on suicide in Bangladesh that will help interested agencies to measure the social and economic burden needed to drive the establishment and implementation of effective suicide prevention programs in the country.

Supplementary Materials: The following are available online at www.mdpi.com/1660-4601/14/9/1032/s1, Table S1: Unadjusted and adjusted analysis of suicide among participants aged 10–17 year olds by socio-demographic and geographical factors, rural Bangladesh. Table S2: Unadjusted and adjusted analysis of attempted suicide among participants aged 10–17 year olds by socio-demographic and geographical factors, rural Bangladesh.

Acknowledgments: We would like to thank Bloomberg Philanthropies for providing the funding to implement the Saving of Lives from Drowning (SoLiD) study. We would also like to thank our local partners, Center for Injury Prevention and Research, Bangladesh (CIPRB) and icddr,b for their invaluable expertise and support in helping us implement the project.

Author Contributions: Shumona Sharmin Salam and Olakunle Alonge conceived the paper, contributed to the data analysis, wrote the initial drafts of the manuscript, and reviewed the final draft for intellectual content. Shams El Arifeen, Dewan Md Emdadul Hoque, Irteja Islam, Shumona Sharmin Salam, and Kamran Ul Baset contributed to the data collection and reviewed the final draft of the manuscript for intellectual content. Shirin Wadhwaniya and Saidur Rahman Mashreky reviewed the final draft of the manuscript for intellectual content. All co-authors provided editing support in finalizing the manuscript.

Conflicts of Interest: The authors declare no conflict of interest. The funding sponsors had no role in the design of the study; in the collection, analyses, or interpretation of data; in the writing of the manuscript, and in the decision to publish the results.

Abbreviations

The following abbreviations are used in this manuscript:

LMIC	Low and Middle Income Countries
HIC	High Income Countries
CIPRB	Center for Injury Prevention and Research, Bangladesh
icddr,b	International Centre for Diarrhoeal Disease Research, Bangladesh (icddr,b)
JHSPH	John's Hopkins School of Public Health
CI	Confidence Interval
IRR	Incidence Rate Ratio
PYO	Person Years Observed

References

1. WHO Estimates for 2000–2012. Available online: http://www.who.int/healthinfo/global_burden_disease/estimates/en/ (accessed on 12 July 2016).
2. WHO Preventing Suicide: A Global Imperative. Available online: http://www.who.int/mental_health/suicide-prevention/world_report_2014/en/ (accessed on 12 July 2016).
3. WHO Disease and Injury Country Estimates. Available online: http://www.who.int/healthinfo/global_burden_disease/estimates_country/en/ (accessed on 7 July 2016).
4. Värnik, P. Suicide in the World. *Int. J. Environ. Res. Public Health* **2012**, *9*, 760–771. [CrossRef] [PubMed]
5. Chen, Y.Y.; Wu, K.C.C.; Yousuf, S.; Yip, P.S.F. Suicide in Asia: Opportunities and Challenges. *Epidemiol. Rev.* **2012**, *34*, 129–144. [CrossRef] [PubMed]
6. The WHO World Mental Health Surveys-Cambridge University Press. Available online: http://www.cambridge.org/catalogue/catalogue.asp?isbn=9780521884198 (accessed on 7 July 2016).
7. Jordans, M.J.; Kaufman, A.; Brenman, N.F.; Adhikari, R.P.; Luitel, N.P.; Tol, W.A.; Komproe, I. Suicide in South Asia: A Scoping Review. *BMC Psychiatry* **2014**, *14*, 1–9. [CrossRef] [PubMed]
8. Wang, C.W.; Chan, C.L.W.; Yip, P.S.F. Suicide Rates in China from 2002 to 2011: An Update. *Soc. Psychiatry Psychiatr. Epidemiol.* **2014**, *49*, 929–941. [CrossRef] [PubMed]
9. Patel, V.; Ramasundarahettige, C.; Vijayakumar, L.; Thakur, J.; Gajalakshmi, V.; Gururaj, G.; Suraweera, W.; Jha, P. Suicide Mortality in India: A Nationally Representative Survey. *Lancet* **2012**, *379*, 2343–2351. [CrossRef]
10. Mashreky, S.R.; Rahman, F.; Rahman, A. Suicide Kills More Than 10,000 People Every Year in Bangladesh. *Arch. Suicide Res.* **2013**, *17*, 387–396. [CrossRef] [PubMed]
11. GHO by Category Suicide Rates-Data by Country. Available online: http://apps.who.int/gho/data/view.main.MHSUICIDEv (accessed on 7 July 2016).
12. Alam, N.; Chowdhury, H.R.; Das, S.C.; Ashraf, A.; Streatfield, P.K. Causes of Death in Two Rural Demographic Surveillance Sites in Bangladesh, 2004–2010: Automated Coding of Verbal Autopsies Using InterVA-4. *Glob. Health Action* **2014**. [CrossRef] [PubMed]
13. Nahar, Q.; Arifeen, S.E.; Jamil, K.; Streatfield, P.K. Causes of Adult Female Deaths in Bangladesh: Findings from Two National Surveys. *BMC Public Health* **2015**. [CrossRef] [PubMed]
14. Hyder, A.A.; Alonge, O.; He, S.; Wadhwaniya, S.; Rahman, F.; Rahman, A.; Arifeen, S.E. Saving of Children's Lives from Drowning Project in Bangladesh. *Am. J. Prev. Med.* **2014**, *47*, 842–845. [CrossRef] [PubMed]
15. Hyder, A.A.; Alonge, O.; He, S.; Wadhwaniya, S.; Rahman, F.; Rahman, A.; Arifeen, S.E. A Framework for Addressing Implementation Gap in Global Drowning Prevention Interventions: Experiences from Bangladesh. *J. Health Popul. Nutr.* **2014**, *32*, 564–576. [PubMed]
16. Alonge, O.; Agarwal, P.; Taleb, A.; Rahman, Q.; Rahman, A.F.; Arifeen, S.E.; Hyder, A. Fatal and Non-Fatal Injury Outcomes: Results from a Purposively Sampled Census of Seven Rural Sub-Districts in Bangladesh. *Lancet Glob. Health* **2017**, *5*, 818–827. [CrossRef]
17. Fontanella, C.A.; Hiance-Steelesmith, D.L.; Phillips, G.S.; Bridge, J.A.; Lester, N.; Sweeney, H.A.; Campo, J.V. Widening Rural-Urban Disparities in Youth Suicides, United States, 1996–2010. *JAMA Pediatr.* **2015**, *169*, 466–473. [CrossRef] [PubMed]
18. Hirsch, J.K. A Review of the Literature on Rural Suicide: Risk and Protective Factors, Incidence, and Prevention. *Crisis* **2006**, *27*, 189–199. [CrossRef] [PubMed]

19. Judd, F.; Cooper, A.M.; Fraser, C.; Davis, J. Rural Suicide—People or Place Effects? *Aust. N.Z. J. Psychiatry* **2006**, *40*, 208–216. [PubMed]
20. Möller-Leimkühler, A.M. The Gender Gap in Suicide and Premature Death or: Why Are Men so Vulnerable? *Eur. Arch. Psychiatry Clin. Neurosci.* **2003**, *253*, 1–8. [CrossRef] [PubMed]
21. Chau, K.; Kabuth, B.; Chau, N. Gender and Family Disparities in Suicide Attempt and Role of Socioeconomic, School, and Health-Related Difficulties in Early Adolescence. *BioMed Res. Int.* **2014**, *2014*, 1–13. [CrossRef] [PubMed]
22. Aggarwal, S. Suicide in India. *Br. Med. Bull.* **2015**, *114*, 127–134. [CrossRef] [PubMed]
23. Parker, G.; Yap, H.L. Suicide in Singapore: A Changing Sex Ratio over the Last Decade. *Singap. Med. J.* **2001**, *42*, 11–14.
24. Hadi, A. Risk Factors of Violent Death in Rural Bangladesh, 1990–1999. *Death Stud* **2005**, *29*, 559–572. [CrossRef] [PubMed]
25. Yusuf, H.R.; Akhter, H.H.; Chowdhury, M.E.; Rochat, R.W. Causes of Death among Women Aged 10–50 Years in Bangladesh, 1996–1997. *J. Health Popul. Nutr.* **2007**, *25*, 302–311. [PubMed]
26. Gipson, J.D.; Hicks, A.L.; Gultiano, S.A. Gendered Differences in the Predictors of Sexual Initiation among Young Adults in Cebu, Philippines. *J. Adolesc. Health Off. Publ. Soc. Adolesc. Med.* **2014**, *54*, 599–605. [CrossRef] [PubMed]
27. Silenzio, V.M.B.; Pena, J.B.; Duberstein, P.R.; Cerel, J.; Knox, K.L. Sexual Orientation and Risk Factors for Suicidal Ideation and Suicide Attempts Among Adolescents and Young Adults. *Am. J. Public Health* **2007**, *97*, 2017–2019. [CrossRef] [PubMed]
28. Masocco, M.; Pompili, M.; Vichi, M.; Vanacore, N.; Lester, D.; Tatarelli, R. Suicide and Marital Status in Italy. *Psychiatr. Q.* **2008**, *79*, 275–285. [CrossRef] [PubMed]
29. Corcoran, P.; Nagar, A. Suicide and Marital Status in Northern Ireland. *Soc. Psychiatry Psychiatr. Epidemiol.* **2009**, *45*, 795–800. [CrossRef] [PubMed]
30. Cutright, P.; Stack, S.; Fernquist, R. Marital Status Integration, Suicide Disapproval, and Societal Integration as Explanations of Marital Status Differences in Female Age-Specific Suicide Rates. *Suicide Life Threat. Behav.* **2007**, *37*, 715–724. [CrossRef] [PubMed]
31. Lorant, V.; Kunst, A.E.; Huisman, M.; Bopp, M.; Mackenbach, J. A European Comparative Study of Marital Status and Socio-Economic Inequalities in Suicide. *Soc. Sci. Med.* **2005**, *60*, 2431–2441. [CrossRef] [PubMed]
32. Khan, M.M. Suicide on the Indian Subcontinent. *Crisis* **2002**, *23*, 104–107. [CrossRef] [PubMed]
33. Khan, M.M. Suicide Prevention and Developing Countries. *J. R. Soc. Med.* **2005**, *98*, 459–463. [CrossRef] [PubMed]
34. Naved, R.T.; Akhtar, N. Spousal Violence against Women and Suicidal Ideation in Bangladesh. *Womens Health Issues* **2008**, *18*, 442–452. [CrossRef] [PubMed]
35. Devries, K.; Watts, C.; Yoshihama, M.; Kiss, L.; Schraiber, L.B.; Deyessa, N.; Heise, L.; Durand, J.; Mbwambo, J.; Jansen, H.; et al. Violence against Women Is Strongly Associated with Suicide Attempts: Evidence from the WHO Multi-Country Study on Women's Health and Domestic Violence against Women. *Soc. Sci. Med.* **2011**, *73*, 79–86. [CrossRef] [PubMed]
36. Pico-Alfonso, M.A.; Garcia-Linares, M.I.; Celda-Navarro, N.; Blasco-Ros, C.; Echeburúa, E.; Martinez, M. The Impact of Physical, Psychological, and Sexual Intimate Male Partner Violence on Women's Mental Health: Depressive Symptoms, Posttraumatic Stress Disorder, State Anxiety, and Suicide. *J. Womens Health* **2006**, *15*, 599–611. [CrossRef] [PubMed]
37. Seedat, S.; Stein, M.B.; Forde, D.R. Association between Physical Partner Violence, Posttraumatic Stress, Childhood Trauma, and Suicide Attempts in a Community Sample of Women. *Violence Vict.* **2005**, *20*, 87–98. [CrossRef] [PubMed]
38. Sudhir Kumar, C.T.; Mohan, R.; Ranjith, G.; Chandrasekaran, R. Gender Differences in Medically Serious Suicide Attempts: A Study from South India. *Psychiatry Res.* **2006**, *144*, 79–86. [CrossRef] [PubMed]
39. Maselko, J.; Patel, V. Why Women Attempt Suicide: The Role of Mental Illness and Social Disadvantage in a Community Cohort Study in India. *J. Epidemiol. Community Health* **2008**, *62*, 817–822. [PubMed]
40. Hawton, K.; Saunders, K.E.; O'Connor, R.C. Self-Harm and Suicide in Adolescents. *Lancet* **2012**, *379*, 2373–2382. [CrossRef]
41. Pitman, A.; Krysinska, K.; Osborn, D.; King, M. Suicide in Young Men. *Lancet* **2012**, *379*, 2383–2392. [CrossRef]

42. Séguin, M.; Renaud, J.; Lesage, A.; Robert, M.; Turecki, G. Youth and Young Adult Suicide: A Study of Life Trajectory. *J. Psychiatr. Res.* **2011**, *45*, 863–870. [CrossRef] [PubMed]
43. Yip, P.S.; Caine, E.; Yousuf, S.; Chang, S.S.; Wu, K.C.C.; Chen, Y.Y. Means Restriction for Suicide Prevention. *Lancet* **2012**, *379*, 2393–2399. [CrossRef]
44. Bálint, L.; Osváth, P.; Rihmer, Z.; Döme, P. Associations between Marital and Educational Status and Risk of Completed Suicide in Hungary. *J. Affect. Disord.* **2016**, *190*, 777–783. [CrossRef] [PubMed]
45. Poorolajal, J.; Rostami, M.; Mahjub, H.; Esmailnasab, N. Completed Suicide and Associated Risk Factors: A Six-Year Population Based Survey. *Arch. Iran. Med.* **2015**, *18*, 39–43. [PubMed]
46. Florentine, J.B.; Crane, C. Suicide Prevention by Limiting Access to Methods: A Review of Theory and Practice. *Soc. Sci. Med.* **2010**, *70*, 1626–1632. [CrossRef] [PubMed]
47. Wu, K.C.C.; Chen, Y.Y.; Yip, P.S.F. Suicide Methods in Asia: Implications in Suicide Prevention. *Int. J. Environ. Res. Public Health* **2012**, *9*, 1135–1158. [CrossRef] [PubMed]
48. Milner, A.; De Leo, D. Suicide Research and Prevention in Developing Countries in Asia and the Pacific. *Bull. World Health Organ.* **2010**, *88*, 795–796. [CrossRef] [PubMed]
49. WHO Reducing Access to Means of Suicide. Available online: http://www.who.int/mental_health/mhgap/evidence/suicide/q7/en/ (accessed on 7 July 2016).
50. Nordentoft, M. Crucial Elements in Suicide Prevention Strategies. *Prog. Neuropsychopharmacol. Biol. Psychiatry* **2011**, *35*, 848–853. [CrossRef] [PubMed]
51. Gunnell, D.; Fernando, R.; Hewagama, M.; Priyangika, W.D.D.; Konradsen, F.; Eddleston, M. The Impact of Pesticide Regulations on Suicide in Sri Lanka. *Int. J. Epidemiol.* **2007**, *36*, 1235–1242. [CrossRef] [PubMed]
52. Matsubayashi, T.; Ueda, M. The Effect of National Suicide Prevention Programs on Suicide Rates in 21 OECD Nations. *Soc. Sci. Med.* **2011**, *73*, 1395–1400. [CrossRef] [PubMed]
53. Fountoulakis, K.N.; Gonda, X.; Rihmer, Z. Suicide Prevention Programs through Community Intervention. *J. Affect. Disord.* **2011**, *130*, 10–16. [CrossRef] [PubMed]

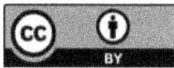

International Journal of
*Environmental Research
and Public Health*

MDPI

Article

Epidemiology of Burns in Rural Bangladesh: An Update

Siran He [1], Olakunle Alonge [1,*], Priyanka Agrawal [1], Shumona Sharmin [2], Irteja Islam [2], Saidur Rahman Mashreky [3] and Shams El Arifeen [2]

[1] Department of International Health, Bloomberg School of Public Health, Johns Hopkins University, Baltimore, MD 21205, USA; siranhe@gmail.com (S.H.); pagrawa6@jhu.edu (P.A.)

[2] International Center for Diarrheal Disease Research, GPO Box 128, Dhaka 1000, Bangladesh; shumona@icddrb.org (S.S.); irteja.islam@icddrb.org (I.I.); shams@icddrb.org (S.E.A.)

[3] Center for Injury Prevention and Research, House # B-162, Road # 23, New DOHS, Mohakhali, Dhaka 1206, Bangladesh; mashreky@ciprb.org

* Correspondence: oalonge1@jhu.edu; Tel.: +1-443-676-4994

Academic Editor: Paul B. Tchounwou

Received: 6 February 2017; Accepted: 31 March 2017; Published: 5 April 2017

Abstract: Each year, approximately 265,000 deaths occur due to burns on a global scale. In Bangladesh, around 173,000 children under 18 sustain a burn injury. Since most epidemiological studies on burn injuries in low and middle-income countries are based on small-scale surveys or hospital records, this study aims to derive burn mortality and morbidity measures and risk factors at a population level in Bangladesh. A household survey was conducted in seven rural sub-districts of Bangladesh in 2013 to assess injury outcomes. Burn injuries were one of the external causes of injury. Epidemiological characteristics and risk factors were described using descriptive as well as univariate and multivariate logistic regression analyses. The overall mortality and morbidity rates were 2 deaths and 528 injuries per 100,000 populations. Females had a higher burn rate. More than 50% of injuries were seen in adults 25 to 64 years of age. Most injuries occurred in the kitchen while preparing food. 88% of all burns occurred due to flame. Children 1 to 4 years of age were four times more likely to sustain burn injuries as compared to infants. Age-targeted interventions, awareness of first aid protocols, and improvement of acute care management would be potential leads to curb death and disability due to burn injuries.

Keywords: burns; epidemiology; Bangladesh; risk factors; low and middle-income countries

1. Introduction

Burns account for approximately 265,000 deaths each year on a global scale, with a huge preponderance in low- and middle-income countries (LMICs) [1]. The death rate due to burns is 11 times higher in LMICs compared to high-income countries (HICs) [2]. Burn injuries mostly occur due to heat transfer from hot liquids (scalding), cooking flames, and sometimes due to exposure to chemicals, electricity, and ionizing radiation [3]. Systematic reviews summarizing studies conducted in the South East Asian subcontinent have identified young age, female gender, poor socioeconomic status and low educational level as major risk factors for burn related injuries and death [4–6]. Some studies have also shown that adolescents and younger adults are at even higher risk of suffering from burn injuries in LMIC, compared to children [7]. Unlike HICs, where preventive measures, first aid and burn care management have been instrumental in curbing burn associated disabilities and fatalities, LMICs are still struggling to address the prevention and management of burn injuries in an efficient manner [8]. In many LMICs, individuals still prefer to treat burn injuries at home (using various mixtures of urine and mud, cow dung, beaten eggs, etc.), thus delaying presentation to a health care facility. Limited resources and dearth of trained personnel in health care facilities also pose major challenges in the appropriate treatment of burn injuries in LMIC [3,8].

Bangladesh is no exception to the burn scenario in South East Asia. Almost 173,000 children in Bangladesh suffered from burn injures in 2003, making it the 5th leading cause of childhood illness in the country [9]. Low socioeconomic status, illiteracy or low educational level, crammed housing spaces, and certain cultural practices are shown to increase risk for burn injuries in LMIC settings [10,11]. Additional risk factors are decreased parental supervision for young children; man-made cotton textiles for clothing, and major female involvement in the kitchen, which explains higher, burn morbidity among females than males [12].

Most data available to indicate the burden of death and disability due to burns in Bangladesh are based on small population-based surveys or hospital registries [5,9]. There is a lack of recent large-scale, population-based data that could describe the burden of burn related injuries in Bangladesh and subsequently identify the issues contributing to burn mortality and morbidity. This paper aims to provide an indication of the epidemiology of mortality and morbidity due to burn injuries across all population demographics in rural Bangladesh and re-evaluate the risk factors associated with the risk of burn related disabilities and fatalities using data available from a large population level baseline survey conducted in rural Bangladesh in 2013.

2. Materials and Methods

A baseline census was conducted in 2013 as part of an injury prevention intervention study, "Saving of Lives from Drowning (SoLiD)" in seven sub-districts (Upazilas) of rural Bangladesh to establish epidemiological characteristics of fatal and non-fatal injuries [13]. The sub-districts were purposively selected because of their higher risk for childhood drowning. The study was implemented with support from two local organizations, Center for Injury Prevention and Research, Bangladesh (CIRPB) and International Center for Diarrheal Disease Research, Bangladesh (icddr,b). The seven selected sub-districts were Raiganj, Sherpur, Manohardi, Matlab South, Matlab North, Daudkandi, and Chandpur Sadar.

The census covered 993 villages, 270,387 households and a population of approximately 1.2 million in 51 Unions of the seven selected sub-districts. Household members were interviewed on a one-on-one basis (typically one member responded on behalf of one household) to retrieve required information using questionnaires developed and tested for the SoLiD study. Data collection was done in two stages. The first round collected general demographic information on all members of a household as well as any record of injury in the past six months and deaths in the past one year. If an individual reported a particular injury mortality or morbidity event during the first round of data collection, an injury specific form was used to obtain detailed information about the injury and death in a second round of data collection. Injury was defined as any external harm resulting from an assault, fall, cut, burn, animal bite, poisoning, transportation of goods and persons, operating machinery, blunt objects, suffocation, and (near) drowning resulting in the loss of one or more days of normal daily activities, schools, or work [13].

All records of fatal and non-fatal burn injuries were retrieved from the primary database for current analysis. All data were de-identified. Fatal and non-fatal burn injuries were analyzed separately. Descriptive analyses were conducted for demographic and socioeconomic characteristics. For burn injuries, summary statistics were presented based on location (home, work place, and others), intention (unintentional, assault, violence or suicide), source of injury (flame, hot liquid/solid, explosive or chemical) and condition of the individual immediately after an injury. Analyses were also carried out to describe the duration and severity of disability due to burn injury. Both mortality and morbidity rates have been reported.

Unadjusted and adjusted logistic regression models were run to describe the risk factors of non-fatal burn injuries in rural Bangladesh. The variables used in the logistic regression models were gender, age, educational level, occupation, marital status and socio-economic status (SES). Unadjusted logistic regression models used each of these variables as a single predictor for non-fatal burn injuries. Adjusted logistic regression model included all variables in one model. Age was categorized into eight groups. Sex was considered as a binary predictor (male as reference group). Educational, occupation and marital status were categorical variables and SES was considered as five ordinal categories (from lowest to highest).

Age was found to modify the odds of having a burn injury with regards to other variables. Thus additional analyses were conducted for children under nine years of age and individuals 10 years and older separately to adjust for the modification. For children under 10 years of age, adjusted logistic regression model considered only age, gender and socio-economic status. (Supplementary Table S1) Results have been presented for individuals above 10 years of age. Estimated odds ratios for the odds of burn injury have been presented.

Ethical Statement

All subjects gave informed consent for inclusion before they participated in the study. The study was conducted in accordance with the Declaration of Helsinki, and the protocol was approved by the Ethics Committee of Johns Hopkins Bloomberg School of Public Health, Center for Injury Prevention and Research, Bangladesh and International Center for Diarrheal Disease and Research, Bangladesh. Ethical approval was provided by the Johns Hopkins Bloomberg School of Public Health (approval code—00004746).

3. Results

The baseline survey covered a total population of 1,169,594 in the seven sub-districts of rural Bangladesh (Table 1). The overall population comprised of about 51% females ($n = 601,919$). About 43% (508,059) of the study population was 25 to 64 years of age. Approximately 35% ($n = 409,923$) received education at primary level. Almost 35% ($n = 408,583$) of the study population was either retired, unemployed, or was housewives. The majority of study participants were married (49%, $n = 571,206$). The population was almost equally distributed across the SES quintiles (lowest 18%, low 19%, middle 20%, high 21% and highest 22%).

Table 1. Socio-demographic characteristics of fatal and non-fatal burns injury patients.

Characteristics	All Population ($N = 1,169,594$)		Fatal Burn Injuries ($N = 25$)		Non-Fatal Burns ($N = 6142$)	
	N	(%)	N (%)	Mortality Rate/1,000,000	N (%)	Morbidity Rate/100,000
Upazila						
Matlab North	265,897	(22.7)	5 (20.0)	18.8	1019 (16.6)	385.3
Matlab South	209,772	(17.9)	3 (12.0)	14.3	1103 (18.0)	528.6
Chadpur Sadar	128,356	(11.0)	0 (0.0)	0	347 (5.7)	271.6
Raiganj	104,357	(8.9)	6 (24.0)	57.5	932 (15.2)	898.2
Sherpur	228,519	(19.5)	6 (24.0)	26.3	1378 (22.4)	606.1
Manohardi	204,319	(17.5)	4 (16.0)	19.6	1150 (18.7)	566.2
Daud Kandi	28,373	(2.4)	1 (4.0)	35.2	213 (3.5)	755.8
Sex						
Male	567,674	(48.5)	2 (8.0)	3.5	1787 (29.1)	316.5
Female	601,919	(51.5)	23 (92.0)	38.2	4355 (70.9)	727.5

Table 1. Cont.

Characteristics	All Population (N = 1,169,594)		Fatal Burn Injuries (N = 25)		Non-Fatal Burns (N = 6142)	
	N	(%)	N (%)	Mortality Rate/1,000,000	N (%)	Morbidity Rate/100,000
Age						
<1 year	22,141	(1.9)	0 (0.0)	0	92 (1.0)	427.4
1–4 years	90,523	(7.7)	0 (0.0)	0	1121 (18.3)	1243.3
5–9 years	139,728	(12.0)	0 (0.0)	0	574 (9.4)	411.1
10–14 years	142,121	(12.2)	1 (4.0)	7.0	377 (6.1)	265.4
15–17 years	62,098	(5.3)	1 (4.0)	16.1	208 (3.4)	335.2
18–24 years	133,534	(11.4)	4 (16.0)	29.9	701 (11.4)	525.5
25–64 years	508,059	(43.4)	6 (24.0)	11.8	2932 (47.7)	579.2
65+ years	71,389	(6.1)	13 (52.0)	182.1	167 (2.7)	244.6
Education						
No education	295,314	(25.3)	17 (68.0)	230.3	1538 (25.0)	526.8
Primary	407,923	(34.9)	4 (16.0)	39.2	1753 (28.5)	430.8
Secondary	289,658	(24.8)	3 (12.0)	41.4	1443 (23.5)	499.3
A levels	45,618	(3.9)	0 (0.0)	0	176 (2.9)	386.7
College	13,526	(1.2)	0 (0.0)	0	38 (0.6)	281.8
Advanced/professional degree	4729	(0.4)	1 (4.0)	845.8	11 (0.2)	234.0
Not applicable (Under 5)	112,664	(9.6)	0 (0.0)	0	1183 (19.3)	1059.2
Occupation						
Agriculture	104,956	(9.0)	1 (4.0)	38.1	234 (3.8)	225.4
Business	61,661	(5.3)	0 (0.0)	0	147 (2.4)	239.7
Skilled labor (Professional)	89,151	(7.6)	1 (4.0)	44.9	263 (4.3)	296.0
Unskilled/domestic (Unskilled)	24,520	(2.1)	0 (0.0)	0	72 (1.2)	295.1
Rickshaw/bus (Transport worker)	17,037	(1.5)	0 (0.0)	0	47 (0.8)	276.6
Students	312,537	(26.7)	1 (4.0)	12.8	922 (15.0)	295.2
Retired/unemployed/housewife	408,583	(35.0)	22 (88.0)	215.4	3059 (49.8)	754.1
Not applicable (children)	144,454	(12.4)	0 (0.0)	0	1369 (22.3)	954.6
Not applicable (others)	5948	(0.5)	0 (0.0)	0	28 (0.5)	484.3
Marital status						
Married	571,206	(48.8)	11 (44.0)	77.0	3358 (54.7)	591.5
Never married	227,319	(19.4)	3 (12.0)	52.8	622 (10.1)	273.9
Divorced	3220	(0.3)	0 (0.0)	0	8 (0.1)	250.2
Widowed	53,096	(4.5)	10 (40.0)	753.4	239 (3.9)	462.8
Separated	2717	(0.2)	0 (0.0)	0	16 (0.3)	592.2
Others (children under 12)	312,035	(26.7)	1 (4.0)	12.8	1899 (30.9)	610.7
SES quintiles						
Lowest	211,601	(18.1)	4 (16.0)	18.9	1254 (20.4)	596.4
Low	218,695	(18.7)	9 (36.0)	41.1	1166 (19.0)	535.8
Middle	238,371	(20.4)	6 (24.0)	25.2	1199 (19.5)	505.6
High	247,716	(21.2)	3 (12.0)	12.1	1258 (20.5)	510.5
Highest	253,210	(21.7)	3 (12.0)	11.9	1265 (20.6)	502.3

3.1. Fatal Burn Mortality Characteristics

There were 25 deaths due to burn injuries among the population surveyed, with a mortality rate of 21 deaths per 1,000,000 people (95% CI: 14–32 per 1,000,000) (Table 1).

Deaths due to burn injuries (92%) were predominantly seen in females, and were significantly higher than deaths in males. Elderly people above 65 years of age bear the burden of burn related deaths. Burns were most commonly seen in individuals who did not have any formal education (68%). Retired or unemployed individuals as well as housewives suffered the highest proportion (88%, N = 22) of burn deaths among other employments. Low (36%) and middle-income (24%) households had the highest burden of fatal burn injuries (Table 1). Deaths due to burns were seen mostly in the winter months (Figure 1). Over half (56%) of the injuries occurred in the kitchen. More than half (52%) of the deaths occurred in the home while 36% occurred in the hospital. Flame injuries (88%) were most common, various sources of flame being cooking fire, heating fire and the kerosene lamp. Two deaths occurred as a result of coming in contact with hot cooking and bathing water (Table 2).

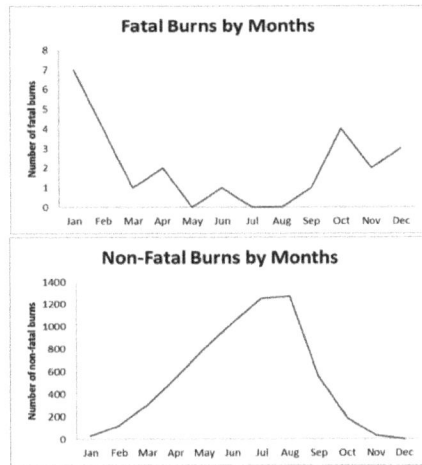

Figure 1. Fatal and non-fatal burn injuries across the months.

Table 2. Distribution of fatal and non-fatal burns injuries.

Characteristics	Fatal Injuries		Non-Fatal Injuries	
	N	(%)	N	(%)
Place of injury				
Bedroom	7	28	273	4.44
Kitchen	14	56	4385	71.39
Veranda	1	4	32	0.52
Yard	3	12	729	11.87
Others	-	-	644	11.78
Item causing injury				
Flame	22	88	1555	25.32
Hot liquid	2	8	3472	56.53
Hot object	0	0	1003	16.33
Explosive	0	0	19	0.31
Chemical	0	0	30	0.49
Other	1	4	63	1.03
Place of death				
Home	13	52		
On the way to hospital [1]	1	4	-	-
Hospital	9	36		
On the road [2]	2	8		

[1] died while being transported to a hospital; [2] did not receive any form of emergency medical assistance.

3.2. Non-Fatal Burn Morbidity Characteristics

A total of 6142 burn related incidents occurred among the approximately 1.2 million people surveyed. The morbidity rate due to burn injuries was 529 injuries per 100,000 populations (95% CI: 517–542 per 100,000). As seen with burn related deaths, more females (71%) had non-fatal burn injuries than males. Higher propensity for burn injuries was seen in children 1 to 4 years of age (18.25%), and adults 25 to 64 years of age (48%), across both sexes (Figure 2). Similar to observations regarding fatal burn injuries, retired or unemployed individuals and housewives had higher prevalence of non-fatal burn injuries, accounting for almost half of all burn related non-fatal outcomes. Almost half of all burn injuries occurred in married people. Non-fatal burn injuries were almost equally distributed across all socioeconomic strata. Unlike deaths due to burns, non-fatal burn injuries occurred mainly in the summer months, with highest propensity in the months of July and August (Figure 1). Almost all burns were unintentional and more than a third (78%) occurred in the kitchen. Contact with hot liquids causing scalds (57%), such as cooking oil appeared to cause the greatest number of burn injuries. Other sources were flame (25%), contact with hot objects (16%), explosives and chemicals. The majority of the cases occurred while preparing food for the household (Table 2).

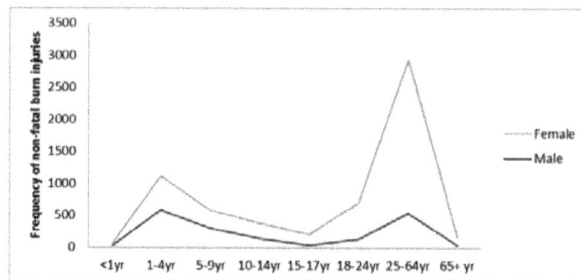

Figure 2. Distribution of Non-fatal burn injuries across age and gender.

An injury severity index was calculated, using indicators such as anatomic and physiologic profiles of an injury, post injury immobility, post-injury hospitalization, surgical treatment, post-injury disability, number of days an individual required assistance, and the number of days lost at work or school. Each of these indicators was classified as binary variables. A principle component analysis (a linear combination of a set of variables to explore the underlying structure of those variables as pertaining to a common factor or factors) was applied to summarize the eight indicators into a single index of severity. The scores for all recorded non-fatal injuries were categorized into tertiles—low, medium and high. Results showed that 71% of burn cases had low severity. Only 4% of the individuals had been severely injured by burns [14] (Table 3).

Table 3. Injury severity index for non-fatal burn injuries.

Injury Severity	Non-Fatal Injuries	
	N	(%)
Low	4283	69.73
Medium	1499	24.41
High	245	3.99

Compared with children 10–14 years of age, adolescents and young adults 15 to 24 years of age had higher odds of sustaining non-fatal burn injuries. Adults 25 to 64 years of age were twice (95% CI: 1.97–2.44) as likely to have non-fatal burn injuries compared with 10–14 years olds. Female participants had more than three times higher chance of burn injuries compared to males (OR = 3.62, 95% CI: 3.36–3.89). The higher the level of education, the lower the risk was for sustaining a non-fatal burn injury. When compared to married people, widowed and never married individuals were at lesser odds of sustaining a burn related injury. Individuals from the lowest socioeconomic level had significantly higher odds to suffer from a burn injury than any other socioeconomic strata (Table 4).

Adjusted logistic regression including all variables (age, sex, education, occupation, marital status and socioeconomic quintiles) showed that the level of education, occupation and socio-economic status was not significantly associated with an amplified risk of burn injury, holding all other factor constant. The ORs did not change meaningfully for age, gender, and marital status while holding other covariates constant. Compared with their respective reference groups, female gender (OR 3.18), and marital status (being married) were found to be at higher odds for non-fatal burn injuries. The lowest SES quintile had higher odds of facing a burn injury when compared with all other four SES quintiles, while adjusting for other covariates (Table 4). Children 1 to 4 years of age were 4.4 (95% CI: 3.37–5.63) times likelier to sustain burn injuries than infants. There was no gender difference in the risk of sustaining a burn injury for children under 9 years of age. Similar association was seen between the risk of sustaining burn injury and socio-economic status among children under 9 years of age as was seen with older individuals, i.e., the higher the socio-economic status, the lower the risk of sustaining a burn injury. Multivariate regression analysis showed increasing age and lower socio-economic status as associated with higher risk of sustaining a burn injury. Gender had no significant association (Supplementary Table S1).

Table 4. Unadjusted and adjusted analysis of non-fatal burn injury by age group, sex, education, occupation, marital status and SES quintiles.

Characteristics	Unadjusted			Adjusted		
	OR	95% CI	*p* Value	OR	95% CI	*p* Value
Age group						
10–14 years	Reference group			Reference group		
15–17 years	1.26	1.07–1.49	<0.001	1.08	0.89–1.32	0.381
18–24 years	1.98	1.75–2.25	<0.001	1.05	0.86–1.29	0.618
25–64 years	2.18	1.97–2.44	<0.001	1.02	0.83–1.27	0.830
65+ years	0.92	0.77–1.11	0.378	0.52	0.39–0.68	<0.001
Sex						
Male						
Female	3.62	3.36–3.89	<0.001	3.18	2.83–3.58	<0.001
Education						
No education						
Primary	0.79	0.73–0.85	<0.001	0.87	0.80–0.94	0.001
Secondary	0.91	0.84–0.98	0.012	0.92	0.84–0.99	0.049
A levels	0.71	0.60–0.82	<0.001	0.86	0.73–1.03	0.105
College	0.51	0.37–0.71	<0.001	0.88	0.49–0.95	0.025
Advanced/professional degree	0.43	0.24–0.76	0.005	0.60	0.33–1.10	0.102
Occupation						
Agriculture						
Business	1.06	0.86–1.29	0.51	1.06	0.87–1.32	0.562
Skilled labor (Professional)	1.31	1.10–1.56	0.003	1.19	0.99–1.43	0.062
Unskilled/domestic (Unskilled)	1.29	0.99–1.69	0.06	1.11	0.85–1.46	0.420
Rickshaw/bus (Transport worker)	1.22	0.89–1.67	0.21	1.19	0.87–1.63	0.269
Students	3.37	2.95–3.85	<0.001	1.12	0.72–1.14	0.407
Retired/unemployed/housewife	1.42	20.79–2.54	0.25	0.91	1.01–1.43	0.035
Marital status						
Married						
Never married	0.46	0.42–0.50	<0.001	0.65	0.55–0.76	<0.001
Divorced	0.42	0.21–0.84	0.02	0.34	0.17–0.67	0.002
Widowed	0.78	0.69–0.89	<0.001	0.68	0.58–0.78	<0.001
Separated	1.00	0.61–1.64	1.00	0.78	0.47–1.28	0.334
Others (children 10–12)	0.41	0.34–0.48	<0.001	0.58	0.45–0.76	<0.001
SES quintiles						
Lowest						
Low	0.94	0.85–1.04	0.01	0.98	0.89–1.08	0.685
Middle	0.93	0.84–1.02	<0.001	0.96	0.87–1.06	0442
High	0.94	0.79–0.92	<0.001	0.98	0.89–1.04	0.745
Highest	0.95	0.78–0.91	<0.001	0.98	0.89–1.08	0.687

4. Discussion

Based on this large-scale cross-sectional data, the mortality rate due to burn injuries was 21 per 1,000,000 populations in rural Bangladesh. The majority of fatalities were seen in children between one and four years of age and the elderly above 65 years of age, as has been reported in previous studies from South Asia [15,16]. Similarly, burn injury mortality was higher among female participants in our study [17–19]. Non-fatal burn injury is quite high in this population (528 people in every 100,000 population).

The study highlighted the disproportionate distribution of non-fatal injuries in select Upazilas in Bangladesh. This finding came as a surprise for the research team as well and on further exploration, no substantial evidence could be found to support the imbalance. This leaves scope for future research work to study these variations, which could possibly generate some best practices from Upazilas to be translated into others with a higher proportion of burn injuries.

Most fatal burn injuries occurred in the winter season. The seasonal variation seen in the distribution of fatal and non-fatal burn injuries can be related to the need for prolonged heating during the winter months. When used for long durations of the night, heat sources such as coal and wood put inhabitants at higher risk of death due to burns [20–22]. Non-fatal injuries displayed different seasonal patterns, and injuries were high during the summer and monsoon months. This is likely attributed to domestic, or occupational activities, such as cooking or working with machinery, that have shorter contact spans and a lower threshold to cause burn deaths. When it comes to location, most burn incidents occurred in the home, mainly in the kitchen. Flames and scalds were the most common cause of burns deaths and non-fatal injuries respectively. Similar results were seen in previous studies from Bangladesh and surrounding countries such as India, Sri Lanka, Pakistan, and Nepal possibly due to the use of unsafe cooking stoves with open fire and lack of safe practice of fuels such as petroleum and butane across regions of South Asia [16,23–28]. A study conducted in Bangladesh covering both urban and rural populations reported electrical burns to be the most common cause of burn injuries [29]. However, since this study was strictly limited to rural regions and did not explore electrical burns, there is scope for further research to tease out the generalized burden of burn injuries in Bangladesh.

Female participants were twice as likely to suffer from burn injuries across all age groups. A study showed that even though boys were more vulnerable to unintentional injuries across all ages, girls were more susceptible to fire related injuries [30]. Similar results as seen in this study were observed in various parts of India, Pakistan, Sri Lanka and Nepal [15,28,31,32]. Cultural and societal norms denote females as majorly responsible for preparing meals in kitchens, which makes them more susceptible to fire injuries. Also, loose clothing, floor level cooking and crammed housing spaces increase risk for sustaining burn injuries among women [11,33].

The lowest socio-economic level was seen to sustain most burn injuries. Another study from Bangladesh showed that children from poor families were almost 3 times more likely to die following a burn injury as compared to children from other socio-economic levels [30]. A systematic review studying various socio-economic factors for the risk of burn injuries reported low income, lack of education, unemployment, crowded and sub-standard living situations, among others to increase risk of burn injuries [34]. In addition, injury severity due to burns has been reported to be higher with reduced SES [35].

This study provides valuable information in terms of analyzing and describing burn injuries in rural Bangladesh. To our knowledge, most studies conducted in LMICs are based on hospital registries and police records. It is likely that a large number of burn mortality and morbidity are not recorded. By conducting a large-scale, household-level survey, this current study is much more representative of the true burden, thus less likely to underestimate the burden of burn injury. Household-level surveys also helped account for bias incurred by facility-based surveys, such as reporting bias, bias in age groups, and bias induced by SES.

Int. J. Environ. Res. Public Health **2017**, *14*, 381

The study also has some limitations. This set of analysis is based on cross-sectional data, therefore cannot support causal association. The covariates selected for regression models were based on program implementation experience and previous literature. This study still cannot pinpoint 'true' causes of burn injuries, but rather, helps identify potential determinants. Second, despite including seven Upazilas, the results still need to be interpreted with caution when it comes to external validity.

However, since the study covered predominantly rural locations in Bangladesh, the results may not be applicable to the urban Bangladeshi population. Studies need to be conducted in both urban and rural settings to measure variations in the burden of mortality and morbidity due to burn injuries.

5. Conclusions

Rural Bangladesh faces a major public health concern in the face of significant prevalence of burn related mortalities and morbidities. Young children and adults are more at risk of sustaining a burn related injury. Females across all age groups are more prone to have a burn injury in their lives. The kitchen environment at homes is most commonly the place of a burn incident. Modifications in a kitchen setup, use of safe cook-stoves and heating sources, complete barricading of the cooking area to prevent contact with children and burn injury prevention educational programs for women are some relevant interventions that may be implemented in rural Bangladesh with involvement from communities to reduce burn related accidents and deaths and thereby reduce the loss of subsequent school and work hours. Age-targeted interventions, awareness of first aid protocols, and improvement of acute care management would also be potential leads to curb death and disability due to burn injuries.

Supplementary Materials: The following are available online at www.mdpi.com/1660-4601/14/4/381/s1, Table S1: Unadjusted and adjusted analysis of non-fatal burn injury by age group, sex and SES quintiles for children under 9 years of age.

Acknowledgments: We would like to thank Bloomberg Philanthropies for providing the funding to implement the SoLiD study. We would also like to thank our local partners, Center for Injury Prevention and Research, Bangladesh and International Center for Diarrheal Disease Research, Bangladeshfor their invaluable expertise and support in helping us implement the project.

Author Contributions: Siran He and Olakunle Alonge conceived the paper, contributed to the data analysis, wrote the initial drafts of the manuscript, and reviewed the final draft for intellectual content. Priyanka Agrawal contributed to the data analysis and wrote the final draft of the manuscript. Shams El Arifeen, Irteja Islam and Shumona Sharmin contributed to the data collection, and reviewed the final draft of the manuscript for intellectual content. All co-authors provided editing support in finalizing the manuscript.

Conflicts of Interest: The authors declare no conflict of interest. The funding sponsors had no role in the design of the study; in the collection, analyses, or interpretation of data; in the writing of the manuscript, and in the decision to publish the results.

Abbreviations

LMIC	low and middle income countries
HIC	high income countries
CIPRB	Center for Injury Prevention and Research, Bangladesh
Icddr,b	International Center for Diarrheal Disease Research, Bangladesh
CI	Confidence Interval
OR	Odds ratio

References

1. World Health Organization Media Center. *Burns*. Available online: http://www.who.int/mediacentre/factsheets/fs365/en/ (accessed on 1 March 2017).
2. Peden, M. *World Report on Child Injury Prevention*; World Health Organization: Geneva, Switzerland, 2008. Available online: https://www.ncbi.nlm.nih.gov/pubmed/?term=Peden%2C+M.+World+report+on+child+injury+prevention (accessed on 19 August 2015).

3. Forjuoh, S.N. Burns in low-and middle-income countries: A review of available literature on descriptive epidemiology, risk factors, treatment and prevention. *Burns* **2006**, *32*, 529–537. [CrossRef] [PubMed]
4. Peck, M.D. Epidemiology of burns throughout the world. Part I: Distribution and risk factors. *Burns* **2011**, *37*, 1087–1100. [CrossRef] [PubMed]
5. Golshan, A.; Patel, C.; Hyder, A.A. A systematic review of the epidemiology of unintentional burn injuries in South Asia. *J. Public Health* **2013**, *35*, 384–396. [CrossRef] [PubMed]
6. Wolf, S.E.; Arnoldo, B.D. The year in burns 2011. *Burns* **2012**, *38*, 1096–1108. [CrossRef] [PubMed]
7. Sharma, M.; Lahoti, B.; Khandelwal, G.; Mathur, R.; Sharma, S.; Laddha, A. Epidemiological trends of pediatric trauma: A single-center study of 791 patients. *J. Indian Assoc. Pediatr. Surg.* **2011**, *16*, 88. [CrossRef] [PubMed]
8. Atiyeh, B.; Masellis, A.; Conte, C. Optimizing burn treatment in developing low-and middle-income countries with limited health care resources (part 1). *Ann. Burns Fire Disasters* **2009**, *22*, 121. [PubMed]
9. Mashreky, S.R.; Rahman, A.; Chowdhury, S.; Giashuddin, S.; Svanström, L.; Linnan, M.; Shafinaz, S.; Uhaa, I.J.; Rahman, F. Epidemiology of childhood burn: Yield of largest community based injury survey in Bangladesh. *Burns* **2008**, *34*, 856–862. [CrossRef] [PubMed]
10. Delgado, J.; Ramirez-Cardich, M.; Gilman, R.H.; Lavarello, R.; Dahodwala, N.; Bazán, A.; Rodriguez, V.; Cama, R.I.; Tovar, M.; Lescano, A. Risk factors for burns in children: Crowding, poverty, and poor maternal education. *Inj. Prev.* **2002**, *8*, 38–41. [CrossRef] [PubMed]
11. Mashreky, S.R.; Rahman, A.; Khan, T.F.; Svanström, L.; Rahman, F. Determinants of childhood burns in rural Bangladesh: A nested case-control study. *Health Policy* **2010**, *96*, 226–230. [CrossRef] [PubMed]
12. Daisy, S.; Mostaque, A.; Bari, S.; Khan, A.; Karim, S.; Quamruzzaman, Q. Socioeconomic and cultural influence in the causation of burns in the urban children of Bangladesh. *J. Burn Care Res.* **2001**, *22*, 269–273. [CrossRef]
13. Hyder, A.A.; Alonge, O.; He, S.; Wadhwaniya, S.; Rahman, F.; Rahman, A.; Arifeen, S.E. Saving of children's lives from drowning project in Bangladesh. *Am. J. Prev. Med.* **2014**, *47*, 842–845. [CrossRef] [PubMed]
14. Alonge, O.; Agrawal, P.; Khatlani, K.; Mashreky, S.R.; Islam, I.; Hyder, A.A. Injury Severity Index for population-based survey, manuscript. (Johns Hopkins University, Baltimore, MD, USA, manuscript in preparation).
15. Lau, Y. An insight into burns in a developing country: A Sri Lankan experience. *Public Health* **2006**, *120*, 958–965. [CrossRef] [PubMed]
16. Gupta, S.; Mahmood, U.; Gurung, S.; Shrestha, S.; Kushner, A.; Nwomeh, B.C.; Charles, A.G. Burns in Nepal: A population based national assessment. *Burns* **2015**, *41*, 1126–1132. [CrossRef] [PubMed]
17. Singh, D.; Singh, A.; Sharma, A.K.; Sodhi, L. Burn mortality in Chandigarh zone: 25 years autopsy experience from a tertiary care hospital of India. *Burns* **1998**, *24*, 150–156. [CrossRef]
18. Batra, A.K. Burn mortality: Recent trends and sociocultural determinants in rural India. *Burns* **2003**, *29*, 270–275. [CrossRef]
19. Laloe, V. Epidemiology and mortality of burns in a general hospital of Eastern Sri Lanka. *Burns* **2002**, *28*, 778–781. [CrossRef]
20. Carroll, S.; Gough, M.; Eadie, P.; McHugh, M.; Edwards, G.; Lawlor, D. A 3-year epidemiological review of burn unit admissions in Dublin, Ireland: 1988–1991. *Burns* **1995**, *21*, 379–382. [CrossRef]
21. El-Badawy, A.; Mabrouk, A.R. Epidemiology of childhood burns in the burn unit of Ain Shams University in Cairo, Egypt. *Burns* **1998**, *24*, 728–732. [CrossRef]
22. Afify, M.M.; Mahmoud, N.F.; El Azzim, G.M.A.; El Desouky, N.A. Fatal burn injuries: A five year retrospective autopsy study in Cairo city, Egypt. *Egypt J. Forensic Sci.* **2012**, *2*, 117–122. [CrossRef]
23. Mashreky, S.R.; Rahman, A.; Chowdhury, S.; Khan, T.; Svanström, L.; Rahman, F. Non-fatal burn is a major cause of illness: Findings from the largest community-based national survey in Bangladesh. *Inj. Prev.* **2009**, *15*, 397–402. [CrossRef] [PubMed]
24. Ahuja, R.B.; Dash, J.K.; Shrivastava, P. A comparative analysis of liquefied petroleum gas (LPG) and kerosene related burns. *Burns* **2011**, *37*, 1403–1410. [CrossRef] [PubMed]
25. Gupta, M.; Gupta, O.; Goil, P. Paediatric burns in Jaipur, India: An epidemiological study. *Burns* **1992**, *18*, 63–67. [CrossRef]
26. Razzak, J.A.; Luby, S.; Laflamme, L.; Chotani, H. Injuries among children in Karachi, Pakistan—What, where and how. *Public Health* **2004**, *118*, 114–120. [CrossRef]

Int. J. Environ. Res. Public Health **2017**, *14*, 381

27. Liu, E.; Khatri, B.; Shakya, Y.; Richard, B. A 3 year prospective audit of burns patients treated at the Western Regional Hospital of Nepal. *Burns* **1998**, *24*, 129–133. [CrossRef]

28. Lama, B.B.; Duke, J.M.; Sharma, N.P.; Thapa, B.; Dahal, P.; Bariya, N.D.; Marston, W.; Wallace, H.J. Intentional burns in Nepal: A comparative study. *Burns* **2015**, *41*, 1306–1314. [CrossRef] [PubMed]

29. Mashreky, S.R.; Rahman, F.; Rahman, A.; Baset, K.U.; Biswas, A.; Hossain, J. Burn injury in Bangladesh: Electrical injury a major contributor. *Int. J. Burns Trauma* **2011**, *1*, 62. [PubMed]

30. Balan, B.; Lingam, L. Unintentional injuries among children in resource poor settings: Where do the fingers point? *Arch. Dis. Child.* **2012**, *97*, 35–38. [CrossRef] [PubMed]

31. Kumar, S.; Ali, W.; Verma, A.K.; Pandey, A.; Rathore, S. Epidemiology and mortality of burns in the Lucknow Region, India—A 5 year study. *Burns* **2013**, *39*, 1599–1605. [CrossRef] [PubMed]

32. Ibran, E.A.; Mirza, F.H.; Memon, A.A.; Farooq, M.Z.; Hassan, M. Mortality associated with burn injury—A cross sectional study from Karachi, Pakistan. *BMC Res. Notes* **2013**, *6*, 545. [CrossRef] [PubMed]

33. Peck, M.D.; Kruger, G.E.; van der Merwe, A.E.; Godakumbura, W.; Ahuja, R.B. Burns and fires from non-electric domestic appliances in low and middle income countries: Part I. The scope of the problem. *Burns* **2008**, *34*, 303–311. [CrossRef] [PubMed]

34. Edelman, L.S. Social and economic factors associated with the risk of burn injury. *Burns* **2007**, *33*, 958–965. [CrossRef] [PubMed]

35. Park, J.O.; Do Shin, S.; Kim, J.; Song, K.J.; Peck, M.D. Association between socioeconomic status and burn injury severity. *Burns* **2009**, *35*, 482–490. [CrossRef] [PubMed]

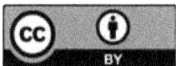

International Journal of
*Environmental Research
and Public Health*

MDPI

Article

Developmental Assessments during Injury Research: Is Enrollment of Very Young Children in Crèches Associated with Better Scores?

Divya Nair [1,2,*], Olakunle Alonge [1], Jena Derakhshani Hamadani [3], Shumona Sharmin Salam [3], Irteja Islam [3] and Adnan A. Hyder [1]

[1] Department of International Health, International Injury Research Unit, Johns Hopkins University Bloomberg School of Public Health, Baltimore, MD 21205, USA; oalonge1@jhu.edu (O.A.); ahyder1@jhu.edu (A.A.H.)

[2] IDinsight, 24/1 Hauz Khas Village, New Delhi 110021, India

[3] International Centre for Diarrhoeal Disease Research, GPO Box 128, Dhaka 1000, Bangladesh; jena@icddrb.org (J.D.H.); shumona@icddrb.org (S.S.S.); irteja.islam@icddrb.org (I.I.)

* Correspondence: dnair1@jhmi.edu; Tel.: +91-997-150-6667

Received: 11 July 2017; Accepted: 18 September 2017; Published: 26 September 2017

Abstract: The Developmental Study is part of a larger intervention on "saving of lives from drowning (SoLiD)" where children were enrolled either into crèches (daycare centers) or playpens to prevent drowning in rural Bangladesh. Sampling ~1000 children between the ages of 9–17 months, we compared problem-solving, communication, motor and personal-social outcomes assessed by the Ages and Stages Questionnaire in the two interventions. After controlling for variables such as home stimulation in multivariate regressions, children in crèches performed about a quarter of a standard deviation better in total scores ($p < 0.10$) and 0.45 standard deviations higher in fine motor skills ($p < 0.05$). Moreover, once the sample was stratified by length of exposure to the intervention, then children in crèches performed significantly better in a number of domains: those enrolled the longest (about 5 months) have higher fine motor (1.47, $p < 0.01$), gross motor (0.40, $p < 0.05$) and personal-social skills (0.95, $p < 0.01$) than children in playpens. In addition, children in crèches with the longer exposure (about 5 months) have significantly higher personal-social and problem-solving scores than those in crèches with minimum exposure. Enrollment in crèches of very young children may be positively associated with psychosocial scores after accounting for important confounding variables.

Keywords: cognitive; psychosocial; crèche; daycare; child development; Bangladesh; Ages and Stages Questionnaire (ASQ); early childhood development (ECD); early childhood care (ECC)

1. Introduction

Early stimulation improves developmental outcomes among young children and these outcomes last over long periods [1–3]. Interventions aimed at children in their early years also yield greater returns than programs that intervene later [4,5]. Early childhood education and care is thus a policy priority given the potential benefits that early cognitive and other stimulation can have on children's problem-solving, communication, motor and personal-social outcomes, and the associated economic and social benefits that may arise at a population level [6].

As such programs become more popular, their designs and contributions to cognitive and behavioral outcomes in varied settings are still uncertain. What types of child-focused programmatic activities will have positive psychosocial outcomes in a particular setting? This is an area of active research [7]. Early child care (ECC) programs in low-and-middle-income countries (LMICs) have only been evaluated recently. These programs have tended to include components on improved nutrition, cognitive stimulation, and cash transfers [8,9]. The cognitive stimulation components have entailed home-visitation programs or counseling sessions where the focus is on at-risk children and training of caregivers [1,5,8,10]. High quality studies that describe ECC programs aimed at large populations of children in institutional settings outside the United States are limited [8,9].

More than a third of children between the ages of 3 and 4 years in LMICs are estimated to have either low cognitive or socio-emotional scores, or both [11]. Bangladesh has been very successful in achieving high primary and secondary enrollment rates, with primary school completion doubling in the last 30 years. However, the country does not have a formalized early childhood development plan. As part of its skill development agenda, and to help equalize learning opportunities, Bangladesh is prioritizing a focus on building cognitive and behavioral skills in early childhood via center-based early learning [12].

ECC provided in out-of-home institutional settings (center-based care) is an unusual offering in low-income settings [9]. In Bangladesh, about 23 percent of children 3–5 years old were attending early childhood education in 2009 [13]. In comparison, in Organization for Economic Co-operation and Development (OECD) countries, about 82 percent of children 3–5 years old were enrolled in pre-primary education in 2011 [14,15]. In addition, about one-third of children between 0–2 years in OECD countries were in some kind of formal care, and these rates are increasing [14,15]. Recognizing the importance of early education, national policy is now shifting towards children between 3–5 years of age (referred to as pre-primary school age). While center-based care in a number of settings has shown high returns [5], child outcomes have largely been found to be associated with the quality of day care centers that form part of the ECC programs [16]. In addition to the low coverage of ECC programs in LMIC settings, the quality of most programs is often poor and the cognitive stimulation involved may not be developmentally appropriate, resulting in poor child outcomes [7].

2. Background on the SoLiD Program

The Saving of Lives from Drowning (SoLiD) project is one of the largest child drowning prevention projects undertaken in a LMIC. It aimed at enrolling around 80,000 children between 9–36 months in 51 unions (the local geographic administrative boundary) and 7 sub-districts in rural Bangladesh. The SoLiD project included two main interventions to prevent childhood drowning in rural Bangladesh. The first involved the use of playpens as a supervisory aid to prevent children 9–36 months from drowning [17,18]. The second intervention involved the enrollment of children 9–36 months into a crèche during the period of the day when they are most at risk of drowning [17]. The quality of execution of the SoLiD project was high, with fidelity to the initial design, and the outcomes on drowning have been promising [17,18].

Children in crèches under the SoLiD project (referred to as "anchal", meaning refuge in Bangla) experienced a wide variety of psychosocial stimulation that was provided to them by crèche mothers who underwent a series of trainings and were given a variety of materials for stimulating the children. It is natural, therefore, to investigate how children enrolled in the creche program gained from such inputs, and whether they experienced improvements in psychosocial outcomes. The goal of this paper is to describe the Developmental Study that was designed to investigate children's psychosocial outcomes and to discuss preliminary results from the baseline survey conducted during 2015. More broadly, the study provides a unique opportunity to examine the early effects of enrollment in crèches among a large group of rural children in a LMIC.

The crèche program under the SoLiD project was designed to be an intensive experience that exposes children (aged 9–36 months and followed up to 48 months) to developmentally appropriate cognitive stimulation. The curriculum was designed by Bangladesh-based child psychologists (to reflect the local context) and included social activities such as story telling, song and dance, and information on personal hygiene and nutrition. Learning included instruction on counting and the rural Bangladesh environment including the geography, flora and fauna. All learning and instruction took place in the local Bangla language. Age-appropriate toys and reading materials based on the local context were also made available.

The crèches operated from 9 a.m. to 1 p.m. six days a week. They were community based, and were run by a crèche mother and her assistant who together supervised 15 to 30 children (a staff–child ratio was about 1:12–1:15). Crèche mothers were trained by master trainers who in turn were trained by the child specialists who designed the curriculum. To ensure local ownership of the crèche, the crèche mother, her assistant, the location of the crèche and other details were decided by a local village committee with support from the project staff. Parent–teacher meetings were regularly organized, and the village committee with support from project staff had oversight over the running of the crèches. Project staff also supervised the activities of the crèche mothers and assistants to assure quality and to provide refresher's training as needed.

The children in the playpens spent an average of 20 min continuously in the playpen per use, and the playpens were used about three times per day. Hence, the total time spent in the playpens was 60 min per day for seven days in a week. The playpens were most often placed inside the house (84% of cases) and less frequently in the yard (14%). Although no program-based psychosocial stimulations were provided for children in the playpens, caregivers/family members were expected to continue to interact and supervise the children while they were in the playpens. Only one child was allowed in a playpen.

The SoLiD project is thus opportune to examine the influence of an ECC program with a focus on stimulation and early developmental outcomes in a low- and middle-income setting. The project aims to monitor psychosocial outcomes for a sample of children under both the crèche and playpen interventions for at least two years. The objective of this paper is to understand the association between an ECC program with a focus on cognitive stimulation and children's psychosocial outcomes in rural Bangladesh within a short timeframe—only a handful of rigorous studies looking at this association come from LMICs (and none are from outside Latin America) [9].

3. Methods

3.1. Design, Participants and Recruitment

This Developmental Study was nested within the larger SoLiD project and involved participants from two (Matlab North and Matlab South) of the seven sub-districts covered in the SoLiD project. Based on a census established for the SoLiD project [17], it identified a total of 7571 children between 9–17 months in March 2015 in these two sub-districts at baseline. Villages were randomly allocated into two areas for the larger SoLiD project: Area 1 had children who received playpens while Area 2 had children being enrolled into the crèches at baseline. The 7571 children across both Areas 1 and 2 were our source population for the developmental study.

In this paper, we describe initial differences that emerged across the two groups. We exploit the design feature that children in both groups experienced varying lengths of exposure as the program was rolled out. Specifically, the difference in dose response is examined, between children randomly enrolled in the playpen (control) and crèche (treatment) groups in relation to how long they were exposed to the interventions.

Eligibility criteria for inclusion in the Developmental Study were that (1) children are between 9–17 months when interviewed; (2) they were enrolled into the SoLiD program on or after 1 January 2015 so that a true baseline is obtained (i.e., exposure to the program was limited); and (3) up to 30 children per village were selected (to prevent an unbalanced design). We calculated a sample size of 1200 (600 in each of Areas 1 and 2) to have a power of 80% to detect a conservative change in psychosocial outcome scores between children under the crèche intervention in Area 2 and those receiving the playpen in Area 1 (this was based on the difference in raw scores and standard deviations observed in other studies in Bangladesh) [19]. We also accounted for the multi-year intervention, correlation between measures over time, and a 20% loss to follow-up while estimating this target sample size. The sample of children was selected using a cluster random sampling technique without replacement. To ensure a total of about 600 children in each arm, we assigned each village a random number in Area 1 and Area 2. We then selected up to 30 children from the villages that were randomly chosen until a total of 600 children was selected from each Area.

3.2. Description of Variables

The Ages and Stages Questionnaire (ASQ-3) is a screening tool developed for children between 1 to 66 months of age [20]. It is widely used in the United States to identify potential developmental delays by parents [21]. The version implemented in this study was translated into Bangla and adapted to the local context by a leading expert in child development who was on the team. The adaptations were made to reflect relevant examples for the Bangladeshi context during the assessment while preserving the original questions from the ASQ. Related to five domains, the questions in the ASQ-3 assessed a child's gross motor, fine motor, communication, problem solving and socioemotional development. The extended version, which consists of 12 questions for each domain, was used; the questions were age-specific and arranged in age bands of two months.

Questions in the ASQ-3 were addressed to parents by trained testers. It took an average of 90 min to conduct an assessment per child. Parents could respond with yes, sometimes, or no (respectively scored as 10, 5 or 0)—12 questions were asked in each domain for a total of 120 points. Table 1 below illustrates each domain with a sample question from the 9-month and 18-month questionnaire. For some questions, the tester actually tested if the child could perform a certain task (indicated by 'test'). In addition, some questions overlapped and were asked across age categories.

Table 1. Sample questions from ASQ-3 for each domain based on age.

Domain	9 Months	18 Months
Communication	If you call your baby when you are out of sight, does she look in the direction of your voice?	When you ask your child to point to her nose, eyes, hair, feet, ears, and so forth, does she correctly point to at least seven body parts?
Gross motor	Does your baby roll from her back to her tummy, getting both arms out from under her?	Does your child jump with both feet leaving the floor at the same time?
Fine motor	Does your baby reach for small things (the size of a peanut/pea/puffed rice) and touch it with her finger or hand?	Does your child use a turning motion with her hand while trying to turn doorknobs, windup toys, twist tops, or screw lids on and off jars?
Problem solving	If a toy falls from her hand while on her back, if she could see the toy, does she try to reach for it?	After she watches you draw a line from the top of the paper to the bottom with a crayon (or pencil or pen), does your child copy you by drawing a single line on the paper in any direction? (Scribbling back and forth does not count as "yes.") (Test)
Personal-social	When in front of a large mirror, does your baby reach out to pat the mirror? (Test)	When playing with either a stuffed animal or a doll, does she pretend to rock it, feed it, change its clothes, put it to bed, and so forth?

A number of relevant control variables were included in the analyses based on a previous study in Bangladesh which suggests that these variables are important measures of health and wellbeing and are relevant for developmental assessment of children in the Bangladesh context [19]: the child's gender, age at testing, Family Care Indicators (FCI), household asset index, head circumference, mother's weight, child's weight, disability, and exposure. The FCI is a standard set of seven questions around items that the child plays with or interacts with in the home. Each response was coded as yes or no and the total number of responses was added up on a scale of seven (where each 'yes' was recorded as one). The questions referred to items that were home-made and bought, but also household materials that were used by the child at home over the last month to play music, color or draw, assist in pretend play, encourage movement, learn shapes, or build blocks. Length of exposure was calculated as time between the date of enrollment of the child into the SoLiD program and the date of interview for the Developmental Study. For the analysis, children were allocated into one of three equal groups based on how much their length of exposure had been (minimum, medium and maximum exposure).

The outcome scores were standardized as z-scores. Unadjusted bivariate associations were first examined between children receiving the playpens and those in crèches for their test scores (both raw and z-scores) and other background characteristics using *t*-test, chi-square and ordinary least square regressions. Ordinary least square regressions were then estimated for each ASQ domain comparing z-scores for children in the crèches with those in the playpens while controlling for relevant characteristics (all control variables were added simultaneously). To account for the sample design, site-specific clustered standard errors (at the village level) and fixed-effect estimates were used to improve estimates. The cluster adjustment was also used to account for the likelihood of children from better off households being located in better neighborhoods/villages, and thus being exposed to better quality teachers, equipment, and lower crèche mother–child ratios within crèches. Sensitivity analyses were done based on length of exposure to the intervention (either crèche or playpen), and the marginal change in outcomes was assessed based on increased exposure.

All testers underwent a two-week training session and inter-observer reliabilities were conducted. Inter-observer reliabilities during data collection using intra-class correlations ranged from 0.93 to 1.0 for different subscales between each of the four testers and the supervisors. In addition, the supervisor conducted (and cross-checked) 10% of the final surveys to ensure comparability and quality control. Participation was voluntary and parents were provided with detailed human consent forms that were explained to them in Bangla. Ethical approval (IRB No. 00004746) for this study was obtained from the Johns Hopkins University and the International Center for Diarrheal Disease Research, Bangladesh Institutional Review Boards.

4. Results

Description of Sample

A total of 1018 children were in the final analytic sample, they were interviewed between April and September 2015 and full data was available for them. Of these, 510 children received just the crèche, while the control group consisted of 508 children who received just the playpen.

Of the original sample of 1435, a total of 417 were not included in the analysis for various reasons. The ASQ score was not accessible for 280 children, socioeconomic measures were not collected for 59 children, and 42 children received both the playpen and crèche—these were all excluded from the analysis. In addition, 21 children came from villages with more than 30 children per village (21 children were thus randomly selected and dropped, and balance across arms was checked to ensure not all children were dropped from one arm). In the final analytic sample, for the treatment group, from Area 2, 80 villages were selected, with village sizes of between 5–80 children. For the control group, from Area 1, 108 villages were selected, with village sizes of between 5–88 children.

The sample was divided into three equal and non-overlapping groups based on length of exposure to the interventions (minimum, average, maximum exposure). The average time between enrollment and interview was found to be 24 days (0–2 months, or "about one month") for children in the minimum exposure category, and it was 72 days (2–4 months, or "about 2.5 months") and 156 days (4–8 months, or "about 5 months") for the average and maximum exposure groups.

In the bivariate analyses, children in the playpen had higher scores than children in the crèche (Table 2). Without adjusting for the control variables, children in crèches had significantly lower scores on all the psychosocial dimensions compared to children receiving playpens. Enrollment in crèches was also associated with significantly lower FCI (at the 1% level) and asset index (at the 10% level). While children in the crèches were not different from children in the playpen in their weight or prevalence of disability, they had slightly lower head circumference (significant at the 5% level) and heavier mothers (significant at 1% level). Children in the crèche also had much lower exposure to the SoLiD intervention (significant at the 1% level). Children in crèches were exposed to crèches for about

52 days on average compared with those in the playpen who have been exposed to playpens for about 115 days (a difference of about two months).

Table 2. Sample characteristics and differences between children in playpen and crèche.

Variables		Playpen (*n* = 508)				Crèche (*n* = 510)				Difference across Interventions? [1]
		Mean	SD	Min	Max	Mean	SD	Min	Max	
Raw Scores	Communication	78.76	18.82	0	120	76.38	19.74	5	120	**
	Gross motor	88.04	22.67	10	120	84.59	23.37	0	120	**
	Fine motor	74.36	18.95	10	120	71.35	19.7	0	120	**
	Personal/social	72.39	23.5	0	120	67.26	23.95	0	120	***
	Problem solving	78.72	20.31	10	120	73.81	20.32	10	120	***
	Total score	392.27	74.13	50	560	373.4	78.79	30	555	***
Z Scores	Communication	0.07	0.99	−4.19	2.61	−0.08	1	−3.38	2.09	**
	Gross motor	0.07	0.96	−3.62	1.65	−0.08	1.04	−4.64	1.65	**
	Fine motor	0.07	0.98	−4.06	2.46	−0.06	1	−3.74	2.33	**
	Personal/social	0.09	1.01	−2.98	2.43	−0.1	1	−2.98	2.43	***
	Problem solving	0.1	1	−3.26	2.4	−0.11	1	−3.37	2.14	***
	Total score	0.11	0.98	−4.72	2.35	−0.1	1.01	−4.37	2.43	***
Controls	Male	55.12				49.8				
	Age	14.31	2.15	9	18	14.07	2.04	9	18	
	FCI	2.25	1.16	0	7	1.96	1.13	0	7	***
	Asset index	0.05	0.97	−2.72	3.7	−0.05	1.03	−3.56	2.88	
	Head circumference	44.57	1.43	40.1	48.3	44.35	1.4	40	48.4	**
	Mother's weight	72.73	26.12	19	99.9	79.21	25.5	24.2	99.9	***
	Child's weight	8.85	1.29	5	15	8.76	1.37	5.2	18.5	
	Exposure (days)	115.37	58.92	−131	243	52.49	46.9	−210	188	***
	Disability	8.76	0.5	6	9	8.77	0.54	5	9	

[1] *** *p* < 0.01, ** *p* < 0.05, Two-sided *t*-tests were conducted for continuous variables and chi-square tests for categorical variables.

In Table 3 below, we display results of ordinary least squares regressions that control for all the variables shown in Table 2. Separate models were run for each domain of the ASQ test. After controlling for relevant characteristics, children in the crèche performed significantly better in fine motors skills than children in the playpen (Table 3). On other dimensions such as communication, gross motor, personal social and problem solving, there were no differences between the children under the different arms. Child's age and weight were significantly associated with ASQ scores for selected domains. Younger children, and children with higher weights were associated with better ASQ scores. The FCI was strongly associated with all domain scores and the total scores; a unit increase in FCI was associated with a 0.4 standard deviation increase in scores (significant at 1% level).

Table 3. Coefficient estimates from multivariate linear regression models, regressing ASQ z-scores in individual and household characteristics.

Variables	(1)	(2)	(3)	(4)	(5)	(6)
ASQ Domain:	Communication	Gross Motor	Fine Motor	Personal/Social	Problem Solving	Total Score
Crèche	0.06	0.27	0.45 **	0.14	−0.06	0.24 *
	(0.22)	(0.22)	(0.17)	(0.16)	(0.16)	(0.13)
Boy	−0.05	0.00	−0.08	−0.04	−0.04	−0.06
	(0.06)	(0.06)	(0.06)	(0.06)	(0.06)	(0.06)
Age	−0.05 ***	−0.08 ***	−0.06 ***	−0.07 ***	−0.07 ***	−0.09 ***
	(0.02)	(0.02)	(0.02)	(0.02)	(0.02)	(0.02)
Family care indicator	0.27 ***	0.22 ***	0.32 ***	0.35 ***	0.33 ***	0.40 ***
	(0.03)	(0.03)	(0.03)	(0.03)	(0.03)	(0.03)
Household asset Index	−0.00	0.02	0.03	0.07 **	0.04	0.04
	(0.04)	(0.04)	(0.04)	(0.03)	(0.04)	(0.04)
Child head circumference	0.01	0.05	0.06 **	0.08 **	0.07 **	0.07 **
	(0.03)	(0.03)	(0.02)	(0.03)	(0.03)	(0.03)

Notes: *** *p* < 0.01, ** *p* < 0.05, * *p* < 0.10; Robust standard errors in parentheses; Village fixed-effects estimated.

Table 3. *Cont.*

Variables	(1)	(2)	(3)	(4)	(5)	(6)
Mother's weight	−0.00	0.01 **	0.00	0.00	0.00	0.00
	(0.00)	(0.00)	(0.00)	(0.00)	(0.00)	(0.00)
Child's weight	0.11 ***	0.09 ***	0.08 ***	0.04	0.00	0.08 ***
	(0.04)	(0.04)	(0.03)	(0.03)	(0.03)	(0.03)
Exposure (Days)	0.00	0.00 **	0.00	0.00	−0.00	0.00
	(0.00)	(0.00)	(0.00)	(0.00)	(0.00)	(0.00)
Disability	0.14	0.33 ***	0.07	0.07	0.11	0.20 **
	(0.09)	(0.09)	(0.08)	(0.08)	(0.08)	(0.09)
Constant	−2.98 **	−6.84 ***	−4.50 ***	−4.80 ***	−4.38 ***	−6.48 ***
	(1.26)	(1.55)	(1.22)	(1.41)	(1.12)	(1.30)
Observations	1018	1018	1018	1018	1018	1018
Number of villages	151	151	151	151	151	151
DF	9.00	9.00	9.00	9.00	9.00	9.00
Adjusted R-square	0.13	0.14	0.17	0.16	0.15	0.26
Rho	0.24	0.22	0.30	0.27	0.25	0.24

Notes: *** $p < 0.01$, ** $p < 0.05$, * $p < 0.10$; Robust standard errors in parentheses; Village fixed-effects estimated.

In the sensitivity analyses, for the adjusted relationship, longer exposure was associated with larger differences in higher scores obtained for children in the crèches (Table 4). Children in crèches who had been "maximally" exposed (about five months) had a 0.63 standard deviation higher total score (significant at the 5% level) than children in the playpen for a similar length of exposure (Table 4). They also had higher fine motor skills (1.47 standard deviations higher, significant at the 1% level), and better gross motor skills (0.40 standard deviations higher, significant at the 5% level). These children are also reported to have better personal/social skills than children in the playpen who have been enrolled for the same amount of time (0.95 standard deviations, significant at the 1% level). Total scores (in column 6) increase from −0.59 to 0.63, and so do all other scores except fine motor skills that fall from 1.79 to 1.47 standard deviations. The largest difference between these two groups is in problem solving, where it is −1.57 among children with the minimum exposure but −0.07 among children with maximum exposure.

Table 4. Coefficient estimate for Crèche intervention from multivariate linear regression models, regressing ASQ z-scores in individual and household characteristics, stratified by length of exposure to intervention.

	Length of Exposure:	Minimum Exposure (About One Month)					
		(1)	(2)	(3)	(4)	(5)	(6)
	ASQ Domain:	Communication	Gross Motor	Fine Motor	Personal/ Social	Problem Solving	Total Score
Panel A	Crèche	−0.19	−0.40	1.79	−1.37	−1.57 **	−0.59
		(0.98)	(1.40)	(1.20)	(0.87)	(0.74)	(1.25)
	Constant	−4.34	−9.46 ***	−8.74 ***	−4.36 *	−5.68 **	−8.74 ***
		(2.71)	(2.31)	(2.85)	(2.57)	(2.81)	(2.66)
	Observations	340	340	340	340	340	340
	Adjusted R-square	0.14	0.16	0.18	0.18	0.19	0.28
	Rho	0.44	0.46	0.65	0.60	0.57	0.44
	Length of exposure:	Medium Exposure (About 2.5 months)					
Panel B	Crèche	−0.90***	0.24	1.11	0.54	1.04 ***	0.60
		(0.23)	(0.24)	(0.88)	(1.37)	(0.23)	(0.62)
	Constant	−2.94	−4.75 *	−3.61 *	−5.30 **	−7.75 ***	−6.82 ***
		(1.94)	(2.68)	(2.06)	(2.47)	(1.75)	(2.19)
	Observations	341	341	341	341	341	341
	Adjusted R-square	0.19	0.16	0.20	0.20	0.21	0.30
	Rho	0.43	0.26	0.38	0.39	0.50	0.28
	Length of exposure:	Maximum Exposure (About 5 months)					
Panel C	Crèche	−0.41	0.40 **	1.47 ***	0.95 ***	−0.07	0.63 **
		(0.34)	(0.18)	(0.18)	(0.34)	(0.17)	(0.24)
	Constant	−2.01	−6.44 **	−4.12 *	−6.74 ***	−0.85	−5.50 ***
		(2.14)	(2.71)	(2.17)	(2.39)	(2.11)	(1.85)
	Observations	337	337	337	337	337	337
	Adjusted R-square	0.10	0.13	0.18	0.17	0.13	0.25
	Rho	0.32	0.31	0.53	0.38	0.31	0.35
Crèche means significantly different across Minimum and Maximum exposure?		No	No	No	Yes	Yes	No

Notes: *** $p < 0.01$, ** $p < 0.05$, * $p < 0.10$; Robust standard errors in parentheses; Village fixed-effects estimated; All variables in Table 1 are included in the regressions.

5. Discussion

Children in crèches had better total ASQ scores and fine motor skills compared to children in the playpen controlling for relevant characteristics, and the longer that children spent in the crèche, the better they performed with respect to their total ASQ scores, gross motor, fine motor, and personal/social scores.

About 30 developing countries had policies on early childhood development by 2005, however, there are no rigorous studies (apart from a few from Latin America) that have looked at the effect of daycare centers on child development outcomes [5,7,9]. The current study begins to address this evidence gap and evaluates the benefits of early center-based care on child psychosocial outcomes.

Given the differences in FCI, household asset index and head circumference at baseline, it appears that children enrolled in crèches had some initial cognitive *disadvantage* as compared with children enrolled in playpens. However, with exposure to cognitive stimulation under the crèche intervention, children had better psychosocial outcomes if they were in the program longer. For all domains assessed, as children spend more time in the program those in the crèches have higher scores over those in the playpens. The contrast is clearest if we examine children who had the least exposure with those who have had the maximum exposure (panels A and C in Table 4), and this is particularly true for the problem-solving domain.

Out-of-home care for very young children in formal settings in low-middle-income countries such as Bangladesh is an unusual experience. In wealthier countries, such institutions are a common location for early childhood learning. In those settings, it has been established that the *quality* of day care centers is most important in determining psychosocial outcomes [7,22]. In the current study, we do not have measures for quality in the current study. We are aware, however, that extensive efforts were made to ensure that the curriculum was designed based on context-relevant expert guidance and that implementation of the program was of high quality [17]. Related to this concern, it is unclear whether this crèche program can be replicated in other settings. The SoLiD program invested significant resources in ensuring the fidelity to initial design and maintaining the quality of implementation. The study is limited in that current estimates are based on a relatively short time frame. While the lack of data on quality of crèches and the short observation period are important limitations, additional information on these variables would improve external validity but the findings remain robust given these limitations. The study also lacked a pure control group (i.e., those without any intervention). However, it is not expected that the ASQ scores of children in the comparison group (those in the playpens) will be different from those who do not receive any intervention given that no program-based psychosocial stimulations were included for the playpen intervention and children spent limited amount of time (less than one hour) in the playpen per day. The study implements an unusual quasi-experimental design involving a much larger number of children (enrolled in a larger number of crèches) and more robust analyses than many other similar studies. Random treatment assignment and sampling of crèche and playpen villages, and including village fixed effects allows us to control for the unobserved differences across villages (differences in socioeconomic status and culture) that may also account for possibly different background characteristics of children in the crèches. Also, the sample for this study was inflated to accommodate 20% loss to follow-up (which is close to the 19% attrition rate observed due to inability to apply the ASQ assessment).

Further assessment will be needed once the children have had additional exposure to the interventions. It is also possible that parents over (under)-estimate their child's ability as measured by the ASQ [23]. However, the design feature of having a treatment and control, and also assessments over time will attenuate this problem. There is no reason to believe that parents of children in crèches respond differently from similar parents of children in playpens with respect to underestimation. However, other information biases are likely, given that the ASQ assessment is based on parental report. For instance, parents of children under the crèches may report better performance because they understand that the crèche is a form of preschool that is expected to improve their children's learning ability. The data collection was conducted without any reference to the interventions, and parents were encouraged to provide objective reports to accurately assess the wellbeing of their children. Moreover, in some studies, parental reports of children's language abilities or their temperament [3] were closely related to their children's scores assessed by testers on language and behavior respectively.

6. Conclusions

The current study provides a unique opportunity for a rigorous examination of the influence of crèches on children's psychosocial outcomes in Bangladesh. The results from this assessment indicate that children in the crèche make greater gains over children in the playpen over a short period. Further research is required to understand if these outcomes are sustained, what kinds of children (for example, by gender, socioeconomic status) gain the most, and also what type of teachers or institutional arrangements for daycare settings are most effective. However, this initial work supports the positive impact of crèches, even though these crèches were primarily designed as a drowning prevention strategy.

Acknowledgments: Bloomberg Philanthropies funded this research.

Author Contributions: Divya Nair conceived and designed the study, conducted the analyses, wrote the drafts, and managed revisions; Olakunle Alonge conceived and designed the study and reviewed the manuscript; Jena Derakhshani Hamadani contributed to the implementation of the study, and reviewed the manuscript; Shumona Sharmin Salam contributed to the implementation of the study, managed the data collection, and reviewed the manuscript; Irteja Islam contributed to the implementation of the study, managed the data collection, and reviewed the manuscript; Adnan A. Hyder conceived and designed the study and reviewed the manuscript.

Conflicts of Interest: The authors declare no conflict of interest.

Abbreviations

The following abbreviations are used in this manuscript:

ASQ	Ages and Stages Questionnaire
ECC	Early Childhood Care
ECD	Early Childhood Development
FCI	Family Care Indicators
LMICs	Low and middle-income countries
OECD	Organization for Economic Co-operation and Development
SoLiD	Saving of Lives from Drowning

References

1. Walker, S.P.; Wachs, T.D.; Gardner, J.M.; Lozoff, B.; Wasserman, G.A.; Pollitt, E.; Carter, J.A.; The International Child Development Steering Group. Child development: Risk factors for adverse outcomes in developing countries. *Lancet* **2007**, *369*, 145–157. [CrossRef]
2. Walker, S.P.; Chang, S.M.; Powell, C.A.; Grantham-McGregor, S.M. Effects of early childhood psychosocial stimulation and nutritional supplementation on cognition and education in growth-stunted Jamaican children: Prospective cohort study. *Lancet* **2005**, *366*, 1804–1807. [CrossRef]
3. Baker-Henningham, H. The role of early childhood education programmes in the promotion of child and adolescent mental health in low- and middle-income countries. *Int. J. Epidemiol.* **2014**, *43*, 407–433. [CrossRef] [PubMed]
4. Carneiro, P.; Heckman, J. *Human Capital Policy*; IZA: Bonn, Germany, 2003.
5. Engle, P.L.; Black, M.M.; Behrman, J.R.; De Mello, M.C.; Gertler, P.J.; Kapiriri, L.; Martorell, R.; Young, M.E.; the International Child Development Steering Group. Strategies to avoid the loss of developmental potential in more than 200 million children in the developing world. *Lancet* **2007**, *369*, 229–242. [CrossRef]
6. Heckman, J.J. Schools, skills, and synapses. *Econ. Inq.* **2008**, *46*, 289–324. [CrossRef] [PubMed]
7. Boo, F.L.; Araujo, M.C.; Tomé, R. *How Is Child Care Quality Measured? A Toolkit*; Inter-American Development Bank: Washington, DC, USA, 2016.

8. Nores, M.; Barnett, W.S. Benefits of early childhood interventions across the world: (Under) Investing in the very young. *Econ. Educ. Rev.* **2010**, *29*, 271–282. [CrossRef]
9. Leroy, J.; Gadsden, P.; Guijarro, M. The Impact of daycare programs on child health, nutrition and development in developing countries: A systematic review. *J. Dev. Effect.* **2012**, *4*, 472–496. [CrossRef]
10. Walker, S.P.; Wachs, T.D.; Grantham-McGregor, S.; Black, M.M.; Nelson, C.A.; Huffman, S.L.; Baker-Henningham, H.; Chang, S.M.; Hamadani, J.D.; Lozoff, B.; et al. Inequality in early childhood: Risk and protective factors for early child development. *Lancet* **2011**, *378*, 1325–1338. [CrossRef]
11. McCoy, D.C.; Peet, E.D.; Ezzati, M.; Danaei, G.; Black, M.M.; Sudfeld, C.R.; Fawzi, W.; Fink, G. Early childhood developmental status in low- and middle-income countries: National, regional, and global prevalence estimates using predictive modeling. *PLoS Med.* **2016**, *13*, e1002034. [CrossRef] [PubMed]
12. World Bank. *Bangladesh Education Sector Review Seeding Fertile Ground: Education That Works for Bangladesh*; World Bank: Washington, DC, USA, 2013.
13. United Nations Children's Emergency Fund. *Early Learning for Development in Bangladesh*; UNICEF: Dhaka, Bangladesh, 2010.
14. Organisation for Economic Co-operation and Development (OECD). *Family Database, Enrolment in CHILDCARE and Pre-School*; OECD: Paris, France, 2015.
15. Laughlin, L. *Who's Minding the Kids? Child Care Arrangements: Spring 2011*; United States Census Bureau: Washington, DC, USA, 2013.
16. Burchinal, M.R.; Peisner-Feinberg, E.; Bryant, D.M.; Clifford, R. Children's social and cognitive development and child-care quality: Testing for differential. *Appl. Dev. Sci.* **2000**, *4*, 149–165. [CrossRef]
17. Hyder, A.A.; Alonge, O.; He, S.; Wadhwaniya, S.; Rahman, F.; Rahman, A.; El Arifeen, S. Saving of children's lives from drowning project in Bangladesh. *Am. J. Prev. Med.* **2014**, *47*, 842–845. [CrossRef] [PubMed]
18. Hyder, A.A.; Alonge, O.; He, S.; Wadhwaniya, S.; Rahman, F.; Rahman, A.; El Arifeen, S. A framework for addressing implementation gap in global drowning prevention interventions: Experiences from Bangladesh. *J. Health Popul. Nutr.* **2014**, *32*, 564–576. [PubMed]
19. Hamadani, J.D.; Huda, S.N.; Khatun, F.; Grantham-McGregor, S.M. Psychosocial stimulation improves the development of undernourished children in rural Bangladesh. *J. Nutr.* **2006**, *136*, 2645–2652. [PubMed]
20. Squires, J.; Bricker, D.; Twombly, E. *Ages & Stages Questionnaires*, 3rd ed.; Brookes Publishing: Baltimore MD, USA, 2009.
21. Rydz, D.; Srour, M.; Oskoui, M.; Marget, N.; Shiller, M.; Birnbaum, R.; Majnemer, A.; Shevell, M.I. Screening for developmental delay in the setting of a community pediatric clinic: A prospective assessment of parent-report questionnaires. *Pediatrics* **2006**, *118*, e1178–e1186. [CrossRef] [PubMed]
22. Peisner-Feinberg, E.S.; Burchinal, M.R.; Clifford, R.M.; Culkin, M.L.; Howes, C.; Kagan, S.L.; Yazejian, N. The relation of preschool child-care quality to children's cognitive and social developmental trajectories through second grade. *Child Dev.* **2001**, *72*, 1534–1553. [CrossRef] [PubMed]
23. Gollenberg, A.L.; Lynch, C.D.; Jackson, L.W.; McGuinness, B.M.; Msall, M.E. Concurrent validity of the parent-completed Ages and Stages Questionnaires, with the Bayley Scales of Infant Development II in a low-risk sample. *Child Care Health Dev.* **2010**, *36*, 485–490. [CrossRef] [PubMed]

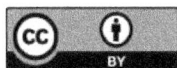

International Journal of
*Environmental Research
and Public Health*

MDPI

Article

Impact of First Aid on Treatment Outcomes for Non-Fatal Injuries in Rural Bangladesh: Findings from an Injury and Demographic Census

Dewan Md Emdadul Hoque [1,*], Md Irteja Islam [1], Shumona Sharmin Salam [1],
Qazi Sadeq-ur Rahman [1], Priyanka Agrawal [2], Aminur Rahman [3], Fazlur Rahman [3],
Shams El-Arifeen [1], Adnan A. Hyder [2] and Olakunle Alonge [2]

[1] Maternal and Child Health Division, International Centre for Diarrheal Diseases Research, GPO Box 128, Dhaka 1000, Bangladesh; irteja.islam@icddrb.org (M.I.I.); shumona@icddrb.org (S.S.S.); qsrahman@icddrb.org (Q.S.-u.R.); shams@icddrb.org (S.E.-A.)

[2] Johns Hopkins International Injury Research Unit, Department of International Health, Johns Hopkins Bloomberg School of Public Health, Baltimore, MD 21205, USA; pagrawa6@jhu.edu (P.A.); ahyder1@jhu.edu (A.A.H.); oalonge1@jhu.edu (O.A.)

[3] Centre for Injury Prevention and Research, House #B-162, Road #23, New DOHS, Mohakhali, Dhaka 1206, Bangladesh; aminur@ciprb.org (A.R.); fazlur@ciprb.org (F.R.)

* Correspondence: emdad@icddrb.org or emdadas@gmail.com

Received: 24 May 2017; Accepted: 9 July 2017; Published: 12 July 2017

Abstract: Non-fatal injuries have a significant impact on disability, productivity, and economic cost, and first-aid can play an important role in improving non-fatal injury outcomes. Data collected from a census conducted as part of a drowning prevention project in Bangladesh was used to quantify the impact of first-aid provided by trained and untrained providers on non-fatal injuries. The census covered approximately 1.2 million people from 7 sub-districts of Bangladesh. Around 10% individuals reported an injury event in the six-month recall period. The most common injuries were falls (39%) and cuts injuries (23.4%). Overall, 81.7% of those with non-fatal injuries received first aid from a provider of whom 79.9% were non-medically trained. Individuals who received first-aid from a medically trained provider had more severe injuries and were 1.28 times more likely to show improvement or recover compared to those who received first-aid from an untrained provider. In Bangladesh, first-aid for non-fatal injuries are primarily provided by untrained providers. Given the large number of untrained providers and the known benefits of first aid to overcome morbidities associated with non-fatal injuries, public health interventions should be designed and implemented to train and improve skills of untrained providers.

Keywords: non-fatal injury; first-aid treatment; medically trained providers; untrained medical providers; rural; Bangladesh

1. Introduction

Injuries are a relatively neglected health issue, [1–4] around 4.7 million people die annually as a result of intentional and unintentional injuries which together account for 8.5% of all deaths globally [5,6]. In 2010, an estimated 11% of the total cause of disability-adjusted life years (DALYs) was attributed to injuries with over 90% of the DALYs lost occurring in low- and middle-income countries (LMICs) [7,8]. Non-fatal injuries occur more often than fatal injuries and have a significant impact on disability, productivity, cost of treatment and rehabilitation [9–11]. It has been forecast that the magnitude of both non-fatal and fatal injuries will decline in high-income countries, but will continue to be a significant cause of death and disability in the developing world over the next 20 years [1,8]. In LMICs, injuries account for about one third of all outpatient hospital visits [7,12]. Despite its overall significance, the burden of injuries in these countries has not yet been fully understood due to lack of population-based data at a country level leading to inadequate preventive efforts, limited resources and ill-equipped healthcare systems to address the issue [1,3,13].

In Bangladesh, sparse data exist to quantify the burden of injuries at the community level. The 2003 Bangladesh Health and Injury Survey (BHIS) indicated that injuries were the greatest killer for children 1 to 18 years of age. According to the BHIS, over 30,000 Bangladeshi children died from injury in 2004, about three children per hour [14]. Drowning, road traffic incidents, falls and burns are among the most common causes of injury in Bangladesh [15,16].

Provision of first aid for injuries is a secondary preventive measures taken immediately after an injury event by trained clinicians and first responders, resulting in better outcomes for injured victims. The International Federation of Red Cross and Red Crescent Societies (IFRC) states that while first aid is by no means a substitute for emergency health services, it is a pivotal primary step for providing effective and rapid interventions to reduce serious injuries and increase the chances of survival [14]. To be most effective, first aid should be provided immediately after the event. For example, effective bystander cardiopulmonary resuscitation (CPR) provided immediately after cardiac arrest can double a person's chance of survival as it helps maintain vital blood flow to the heart and brain [14]. Also, the immediate application of running cold water for 20 min, can stop the burn process and positively affect the outcome of burns [17,18]. Studies conducted in developed countries on non-fatal injuries have reported first aid to play a significant role in reducing mortality rates [19]. In developing countries, several studies have shown that first aid given by an untrained provider (e.g., caregiver, bystander) or a trained provider is increasingly essential to reduce mortality as well as severity of injuries [19–22]. Research on severe non-fatal injuries such as burns, blunt trauma and road traffic incidents in high-income settings has found significant reduction in mortality rates when first aid was applied [19,22,23]. Despite the large burden of injuries in LMICs and the importance of first aid in decreasing injury severity and increasing survival, there is a dearth of research in LMICs like Bangladesh around the subject [1,3]. Moreover, the few available studies in LMICs are hospital-based and suggest that a significant proportion of patients with non-fatal injury events did not receive first aid treatment from any health care facility [24]. Therefore, the objective of this study was to quantify the impact of first aid provided by trained and untrained providers on severe, non-fatal injuries in rural Bangladesh using population-based data collected from a baseline census conducted in 2013 as part of a drowning prevention study.

2. Materials and Methods

2.1. Study Design, Area and Population

This paper is based on data collected as part of a large-scale implementation study, "Saving of children's Lives from Drowning" (SOLID) project [25,26]. A cross-sectional baseline census was conducted over a period of six months (June to November 2013) prior to implementing a package of drowning prevention interventions in seven rural sub-districts of Bangladesh. The baseline census covered approximately 1.16 million people (based on the 2011 Bangladesh National Census) across 51 unions from Matlab North, Matlab South, Daudkandi, Chandpur Sadar, Manohardi, Raiganj and Sherpur Sadar. Unions are the lowest administrative unit of local government in Bangladesh [27].

2.2. Questionnaire and Data Collection

The baseline census collected information on socio-demographic details, injury events, first aid practices and health care seeking behaviors for all injury events and outcomes on all populations in selected sub-districts. Data was collected using a structured, pre-tested questionnaire and consisted of seven modules. Specific questions related to first aid practices and health care seeking behaviors were considered in the injury morbidity (module V) and injury mortality (module VI) modules. All non-fatal injury related information was collected over a six-month recall period; however, deaths were collected over a one-year recall period. Face-to-face interviews were conducted with the household head or any household member 18 years and older to collect all required information. All the tools were written in English and translated to Bangla and written informed consent was obtained from all respondents [27]. The survey was implemented such that the "don't know" where later confirmed as a "no" based on the follow-up questions asked by the interviewer. The instruction that was given to the interviewer was that they needed to clarify if any treatment was obtained by the injured person, and all those who responded no or don't know were asked some follow-up questions such as if the injured was taken to a hospital, or healthcare provider, or if any interventions was administered to help ascertain that they in fact did not receive any treatment.

Non-fatal injury was defined as "any household member who sought treatment or lost at least one working day or could not go to the school for at least one day due to any of injury events". First-aid treatment was defined as "any household member who received emergency care (from medically trained or untrained provider) immediately after the injury and prior to full medical treatment, if treatment was sought". Health care seeking behavior was defined as "any household member who sought first aid treatment or any type of surgical or medical intervention either from trained health care provider or untrained provider". Registered medical doctors and nurses were considered as trained providers whereas any other person, such as friends, peers, village doctors, or relatives were considered as untrained providers. Information on the treatment outcomes after first aid was also obtained. For each participant reporting an injury event, an injury severity score was calculated based on principal component analysis on eight variables—anatomic and physiologic profiles of an injury, post injury immobility, post-injury hospitalization, surgical treatment, post-injury disability, number of days an individual required assistance, and the number of days lost at work or school. The injury severity scores were categorized into severity tertiles that correspond with low, medium and high severity categories [27]. In addition, treatment outcomes were described for all non-fatal hospitalized injuries, and these were categorized into no improvement, recovering or fully functional and anatomic recovery. 'Fully recovered' is defined as anybody who has reported to have regained full physiological and anatomical functionality of the part of the body that was injured. If the physiological and anatomical functionality is better than when the injury took place, but not at the level experienced prior to the injury, it was classified as 'improving'. If the physiological and anatomically functionality remains at the same level as it was during the injury, then it was categorized as 'no improvement'. This was a self-reported information obtained based on the perception of the injured individuals regarding their state irrespective of their injury severity or whether they had received first aid or not.

2.3. Statistical Method and Analyses

Counts and frequencies of non-fatal injuries were calculated and categorized under each injury severity categories: low, medium and high severity. The counts and frequencies under each injury severity categories were further described by whether the individuals received first aid or not. Counts and frequencies were calculated for those that received first aid, and these were described by age, sex, external causes of injury, occupation, educational attainment, geographical area and type of provider (medically trained compared to untrained).

For all injuries categorized under the high severity category and for which first aid was provided, the association between treatment outcomes and types of service provider were assessed using multivariate logistic regression models, and adjusted for key covariates including the external causes, educational level, occupation, wealth quintile, age, sex and geographic area of each household member. All estimations were reported as odds ratios (OR), with their respective 95% confidence intervals (CI). Variable construction and estimations were done with statistical software STATA V.13 (Stata Corp., College Station, TX, USA).

2.4. Ethical Approval

Ethical approval for the study was obtained from the Institutional Review Boards of the Johns Hopkins Bloomberg School of Public Health, USA; International Centre for Diarrheal Disease Research, Bangladesh and the Centre for Injury Prevention Research, Bangladesh (ethical approval code: 00004746).

3. Results

Overall, 21.6% of the respondents were less than 10 years of age, 72.6% were 10 to 65 years of age and only 5.9% were more than 65 years old (Table 1) [27]. Around 60% of the respondents had received at least primary or secondary education. Around 78% were unemployed of which 27% were students; employed individuals were involved in agricultural activities (9%), skilled work (7.7%) and business (5.3%). The contribution of respondents by sub-district was Matlab North (22.8%), Matlab South (18.2%), Chandpur Sadar (11.0%) of Chandpur district, Sherpur Sadar (19.4%) of Sherpur district, Manohardi (17.3%) of Narshingdi district and Raiganj (8.8%) of Sirajgonj district.

A total of 1,159,966 individuals were included in the study of which 8.7% had sustained at least one injury in the six months preceding the date of the interview (Table 2). The total number of non-fatal injury events recorded were 115,385, of which 6.5% (n = 76,469) were in the low severity tertile; 2.1% (n = 24,018) in medium and 1.3% (n = 14,898) were included in the high injury severity tertile.

Table 1. Socio-demographic characteristics of the rural population from seven sub-districts of Bangladesh, 2013.

Characteristics	n = 1,159,966	%
Age (in years)		
<10 years	250,173	21.6
10–14 years	141,725	12.2
15–17 years	61,939	5.3
18–24 years	133,161	11.5
25–64 years	504,850	43.5
≥65 years	68,118	5.9
Sex		
Male	562,721	48.5
Female	597,245	51.5
Education (n = 1,159,815)		
No education	291,021	25.1
Primary complete (5 years)	405,633	35.0
Secondary complete (10 years)	288,465	24.9
Secondary+	63,595	5.5
Under 5 children	111,101	9.6
Occupation (n = 1,159,230)		
Skilled labor (Professional)	88,645	7.6
Agriculture	103,387	8.9
Business	61,166	5.3
Unskilled/domestic (Unskilled)	24,327	2.1
Rickshaw/bus (Transport worker)	16,921	1.5
Students	311,587	26.9
Retired/unemployed/housewife	404,765	34.9
Not applicable (children & others)	148,432	12.8
Marital Status		
Married (Reference)	566,268	48.8
Never Married	226,666	19.5
Widowed/Divorced/Separated	57,390	4.9
Not applicable	309,642	26.7

Table 1. *Cont.*

Characteristics	n = 1,159,966	%
Wealth quintile		
Lowest	209,500	18.1
Low	216,906	18.7
Middle	236,547	20.4
High	245,820	21.2
Highest	251,191	21.6
Sub-district		
Matlab North	264,315	22.8
Matlab South	208,443	18.0
Chandpur Sadar	127,743	11.0
Raiganj	102,526	8.8
Sherpur Sadar	226,677	20.0
Manohardi	202,092	17.4
Daudkandi	28,170	2.4
District		
Chandpur/comilla	628,671	54.2
Sirajganj	102,526	8.8
Sherpur	226,677	19.5
Narshingdi	202,092	17.4

Table 2. Number of individuals and non-fatal injury events by injury severity, 2013.

Characteristics	Number of Injury Events (n = 1,173,974)		Number of Individuals (n = 1,159,966)	
	n	%	n	%
No Injury	1,058,589	90.17	1,058,589	91.26
Non-Fatal Injury severity	115,385	9.83	101,377	8.74
Low	76,469	6.51	66,430	5.73
Medium	24,018	2.05	21,453	1.85
High	14,898	1.27	13,494	1.16

First aid from any provider was received for 81.7% (*n* = 94,232) of all recorded non-fatal injury events and was slightly more frequent low (82.5%) or medium (81.5%) severity injuries compared to injuries that were very severe (77.9%) (*p* value < 0.001) (Table 3). The proportion of people receiving first aid from medically trained providers increased as the severity of the injury increased (*p* value < 0.001). About 7.1% of those who received first aid from a medically trained provider were in the high severity category, as compared to only 1.5% in the low severity category. The situation was reverse for those receiving first aid from a non-medically trained provider −81.4% of those with low severity injury sought care from a non-medical provider compared to 72.9% of high severity injuries. The difference in obtaining first aid from both kinds of provider by severity category was found to be significant (Table 3).

Table 3. Percentage of non-fatal injury events that received first-aid according to injury severity categories, 2013.

Severity Category	Received First Aid n (%) [1]		Received First Aid from Medically Trained Provider n (%) [1]		Received First Aid from Non-Medically Trained Providers n (%) [1]	
	Yes	No	Yes	No	Yes	No
Low	63,058 (82.5)	13,411 (17.5)	1175 (1.5)	75,294 (98.5)	62,282 (81.4)	14,187 (18.6)
Medium	19,572 (81.5)	4446 (18.5)	756 (3.1)	23,262 (96.9)	19,049 (79.3)	4969 (20.7)
High	11,602 (77.9)	3296 (22.1)	1053 (7.1)	13,845 (92.9)	10,858 (72.9)	4040 (27.1)
Total	94,232 (81.7)	21,153 (18.3)	2984 (2.6)	112,401 (97.4)	92,189 (79.9)	23,196 (20.1)

[1] All significant at *p*-value of <0.001.

Among all injury severity categories, receiving first aid was more common for fall injuries (39%), followed by cuts (23.4%) and injuries sustained from a blunt object (9.4%). Among those who received first aid, just over half (52%) were aged 25–64 years, and 59.3% residents were from Chandpur and Comilla districts (Table 4).

Table 4. The percentage of non-fatal injury events that received first aid by type of provider, injury mechanism, socio-demographic and geographical factors among different non-fatal injury severity categories.

Characteristics	Injury Severity Tertiles			
	Low *n* (%)	Medium *n* (%)	High *n* (%)	Total *n* (%)
n (Number of injury events that received first aid)	63,058 (100)	19,572 (100)	11,602 (100)	94,232 (100)
External cause of injury				
Attempted suicide	18 (0.0)	2 (0.0)	19 (0.2)	39 (0.0)
Transport injury	3596 (5.7)	2079 (10.6)	1379 (11.9)	7054 (7.5)
Violence	1087 (1.7)	486 (2.5)	790 (6.8)	2363 (2.5)
Fall	22,685 (36.0)	7793 (39.8)	6288 (54.2)	36,766 (39.0)
Cut injury	16,815 (26.7)	4508 (23.0)	732 (6.3)	22,055 (23.4)
Burn	3948 (6.3)	1386 (7.1)	200 (1.7)	5534 (5.9)
Drowning	1778 (2.8)	59 (0.3)	600 (5.2)	2437 (2.6)
Unintentional poisoning	19 (0.0)	8 (0.0)	39 (0.3)	66 (0.1)
Machine injury	566 (0.9)	270 (1.4)	133 (1.2)	969 (1.0)
Electrocution	401 (0.6)	74 (0.4)	190 (1.6)	665 (0.7)
Animal bite injury	5974 (9.5)	870 (4.5)	402 (3.5)	7246 (7.7)
Injury by blunt object	6064 (9.6)	2029 (10.4)	799 (6.9)	8892 (9.4)
Suffocation	107 (0.2)	8 (0.0)	31 (0.3)	146 (0.2)
Age (in years)				
<10 years	12,865 (20.4)	3028 (15.5)	2428 (20.9)	18,321(19.4)
10–14 years	6324 (10.0)	1729 (8.8)	977 (8.4)	9030 (9.6)
15–17 years	2530 (4.0)	788 (4.0)	375 (3.2)	3693 (3.9)
18–24 years	5412 (8.6)	1624 (8.3)	787 (6.8)	7823 (8.3)
25–64 years	32,259 (51.2)	10,788 (55.1)	5936 (51.2)	48,983 (52.0)
≥65 years	3668 (5.8)	1615 (8.3)	1099 (9.5)	6382 (6.8)
Sub-district				
Matlab North	13,109 (20.8)	5592 (28.6)	3011 (26.0)	21,712 (23.0)
Matlab South	14,282 (22.7)	4356 (22.3)	2828 (24.4)	21,466 (22.8)
Chandpur Sadar	4416 (7.0)	2642 (13.5)	1487 (12.8)	8545 (9.1)
Raiganj	9507 (15.1)	1735 (8.9)	1233 (10.6)	12,475 (13.2)
Sherpur	9725 (15.4)	2026 (10.4)	1467 (12.6)	13,218 (14.0)
Manohardi	9077 (14.4)	2362 (12.1)	1211 (10.4)	12,650 (13.4)
Daud Kandi	2942 (4.7)	859 (4.4)	365 (3.2)	4166 (4.4)
District				
Chandpur/Comilla	34,749 (55.1)	13,449 (68.7)	7691 (66.3)	55,889 (59.3)
Sirajgonj	9507 (15.1)	1735 (8.9)	1233 (10.6)	12,475 (13.2)
Sherpur	9725 (15.4)	2026 (10.4)	1467 (12.6)	13,218 (14.0)
Narshingdi	9077 (14.4)	2362 (12.1)	1211 (10.4)	12,650 (13.4)

The hospitalized non-fatal injured persons of high severity who received first aid were either improving (62.6%) or had recovered (33.2%). The largest proportion of patients for all the outcomes were 25 to 64 years of age and were male. Among the 108 severe non-fatal injury patients that reported no improvement, only 8.3% saw a medically trained provider, while about two-thirds (65.7%) received first aid treatment from an untrained provider. Of those cases with no improvement, almost two-third was reported to have sustained injuries due to falls and road traffic incidents. Among the 1582 patients that were reportedly improving, 930 (58.8%) went to untrained provider for treatment and only 234 (14.8%) received first aid treatment from medically trained providers. Falls (29.7%), transport injury

(27.4%) and violence (21.4%) were the commonest mechanisms of injury reported among this group. Of the 838 participants who recovered, only 160 (19.1%) received treatment from medically trained provider and 479 (57.2%) went to untrained provider for first-aid treatment. The most common causes of severe non-fatal injury among those who recovered were transport injuries (24.2%), falls (24.1%) and violence (23.2%) (Table 5).

Table 5. The distribution of treatment outcomes by injury mechanism, socio-demographic and geographical factors among severe non-fatal hospitalized injury patients.

Characteristics	Treatment Outcome					
	No Improvement		Improving		Recovered	
	n	%	*n*	%	*n*	%
Severe non-fatal hospitalized injury events who received first aid	108	4.3	1582	62.6	838	33.2
Received first aid from Medically trained provider						
No	99	91.7	1348	85.2	678	80.9
Yes	9	8.3	234	14.8	160	19.1
Received first aid from non-medically trained providers						
No	37	34.3	652	41.2	359	42.8
Yes	71	65.7	930	58.8	479	57.2
External cause of severe non-fatal injury						
Attempted suicide	0	0.0	9	0.6	6	0.7
Transport injury	33	30.6	433	27.4	203	24.2
Violence	15	13.9	339	21.4	194	23.2
Fall	36	33.3	470	29.7	202	24.1
Cut injury	4	3.7	91	5.8	68	8.1
Burn	3	2.8	37	2.3	23	2.7
Drowning	0	0.0	14	0.9	17	2.0
Unintentional poisoning	0	0.0	7	0.4	7	0.8
Machine injury	2	1.9	31	2.0	18	2.1
Electrocution	2	1.9	25	1.6	21	2.5
Animal bite injury	2	1.9	38	2.4	29	3.5
Injury by blunt object	11	10.2	87	5.5	49	5.8
Suffocation	0	0.0	1	0.1	1	0.1
Age (in years)						
<10 years	6	5.6	168	10.6	113	13.5
10–14 years	5	4.6	94	5.9	53	6.3
15–17 years	7	6.5	68	4.3	39	4.7
18–24 years	9	8.3	165	10.4	96	11.5
25–64 years	66	61.1	946	59.8	485	57.9
≥65 years	15	13.9	141	8.9	52	6.2
Sex						
Male	71	65.7	1099	69.5	598	71.4
Female	37	34.3	483	30.5	240	28.6
Sub-district						
Matlab North	25	23.1	384	24.3	224	26.7
Matlab South	15	13.9	411	26.0	96	11.5
Chandpur Sadar	22	20.4	243	15.4	85	10.1
Raiganj	27	25.0	103	6.5	87	10.4
Sherpur	8	7.4	227	14.3	189	22.6
Manohardi	8	7.4	180	11.4	151	18.0
Daudkandi	3	2.8	34	2.1	6	0.7
District						
Chandpur/Comilla	65	60.2	1072	67.8	411	49.0
Sirajgonj	27	25.0	103	6.5	87	10.4
Sherpur	8	7.4	227	14.3	189	22.6
Narshingdi	8	7.4	180	11.4	151	18.0

Those non-fatal injury cases that had received first aid from a medically trained provider were more likely to recover or were in the process of improvement compared to those who received first aid from an untrained provider (OR 1.28; 95% CI 1.02–1.61) (Table 6). The chances of recovery were significantly higher among patients in Sherpur (OR 2.05; 95% CI 1.62–2.60) and Narshingdi (OR 1.98; 95% CI 1.55–2.54) districts, as compared to Chandpur/Comilla districts. However, the odds of recovery were less among those who received surgical intervention (OR 0.55; 95% CI 0.45–0.68), participants aged 25 years of age and older compared to children 10 years of age or less (OR 0.55; 95% CI 0.33–0.92) and among retired person/housewives compared to skilled laborers (OR 0.71; 95% CI 0.51–0.99).

Table 6. Multivariate analysis of treatment outcomes by trained provider among severe non-fatal hospitalized injuries.

| Characteristics | Treatment Outcome (1 = Recovered/Improving; 0 = No Improvement) | | | |
| | Unadjusted | | Adjusted | |
	OR	95% CI	OR	95% CI
Received first aid from trained provider				
Yes	1.44 *	1.16–1.79	1.28 *	1.02–1.61
No	Reference group		Reference group	
Surgical intervention				
Yes	0.52 *	0.43–0.63	0.55 *	0.45–0.68
No	Reference group		Reference group	
External cause of severe non-fatal injury				
Attempted suicide	Reference group		Reference group	
Transport injury	0.6	0.22–1.64	0.613	0.22–1.72
Violence	0.78	0.28–2.14	0.902	0.32–2.52
Fall	0.55	0.20–1.52	0.652	0.23–1.83
Cut injury	1.00	0.35–2.85	0.975	0.34–2.82
Burn	0.77	0.25–2.36	0.650	0.21–2.05
Drowning	1.74	0.51–5.87	1.499	0.42–5.34
Unintentional poisoning	1.45	0.34–6.06	1.435	0.33–6.19
Machine injury	0.75	0.24–2.36	0.904	0.28–2.91
Electrocution	1.04	0.33–3.28	0.953	0.30–3.07
Animal bite injury	1.01	0.33–3.03	0.906	0.29–2.80
Injury by blunt object	0.63	0.22–1.80	0.776	0.26–2.28
Suffocation	1.45	0.08–26.26	1.406	0.08–26.17
Age (in years)				
<10 years	Reference group		Reference group	
10–14 years	0.81	0.54–1.21	0.78	0.48–1.25
15–17 years	0.73	0.47–1.14	0.68	0.39–1.19
18–24 years	0.83	0.59–1.16	0.73	0.43–1.23
25–64 years	0.71 *	0.55–0.92	0.55 **	0.33–0.92
≥65 years	0.48 *	0.33–0.69	0.45 *	0.25–0.81
Sex				
Male	Reference group		Reference group	
Female	0.89	0.74–1.06	1.13	0.89–1.45
Wealth quintile				
Lowest	Reference group		Reference group	
Low	1.00	0.77–1.29	1.06	0.81–1.39
Middle	1.07	0.83–1.38	1.15	0.88–1.50
High	0.86	0.66–1.11	0.95	0.73–1.25
Highest	0.89	0.68–1.16	1.08	0.81–1.44

Table 6. *Cont.*

| Characteristics | Treatment Outcome (1 = Recovered/Improving; 0 = No Improvement) | | | |
| | Unadjusted | | Adjusted | |
	OR	95% CI	OR	95% CI
District				
Chandpur/comilla	Reference group		Reference group	
Sirajganj	1.38 **	1.02–1.87	1.29	0.94–1.78
Sherpur	2.16 *	1.74–2.69	2.05 *	1.62–2.60
Narshingdi	2.14 *	1.69–2.71	1.98 *	1.55–2.54
Occupation				
Skilled labor (Professional)	Reference group		Reference group	
Agriculture	1.23	0.92–1.65	1.18	0.86–1.60
Business	0.97	0.68–1.37	0.97	0.68–1.39
Unskilled/domestic (Unskilled)	1.04	0.66–1.62	0.99	0.62–1.56
Rickshaw/bus (Transport worker)	1.32	0.87–2.01	1.30	0.84–2.01
Students	1.07	0.80–1.44	0.75	0.48–1.18
Retired/unemployed/housewife	0.71 **	0.55–0.93	0.71 **	0.51–0.99
Not applicable (children & others)	1.33	0.92–1.92	0.66	0.32–1.38
Education				
No education	Reference group		Reference group	
Primary	0.98	0.80–1.20	0.97	0.78–1.21
Secondary	0.92	0.74–1.14	0.96	0.74–1.24
A levels/college/Advanced/ Professional Degree	0.85	0.58–1.25	0.95	0.61–1.48
Not applicable (U5 children)	1.36	0.94–1.98	1.09	0.51–2.30

$* p < 0.01, ** p < 0.05.$

Treatment outcome was not significantly different for those who received first aid from a non medically trained provider, as compared with those who did not receive first aid (Table 7).

Table 7. Multivariate analysis of treatment outcomes by un-trained provider among severe non-fatal hospitalised injuries.

| Characteristics | Treatment Outcome (1 = Recovered/Improving; 0 = No Improvement) | | | |
| | Unadjusted | | Adjusted | |
	OR	95% CI	OR	95% CI
Receiver first aid from untrained Provider				
Yes	0.89	0.76–1.05	0.90	0.76–1.06
No	Reference group		Reference group	
Surgical intervention				
Yes	0.52 *	0.43–0.63	0.55 *	0.45–0.67
No	Reference group		Reference group	
External cause of severe non-fatal injury				
Attempted suicide/suicide	Reference group		Reference group	
Transport injury	0.60	0.22–1.64	0.611	0.21–1.71
Violence	0.78	0.28–2.14	0.896	0.31–2.51
Fall	0.55	0.20–1.52	0.657	0.23–1.84
Cut injury	1.00	0.35–2.85	0.990	0.34–2.86
Burn	0.77	0.25–2.36	0.657	0.20–2.07
Drowning	1.74	0.51–5.87	1.558	0.43–5.55
Unintentional poisoning	1.45	0.34–6.06	1.530	0.35–6.58
Machine injury	0.75	0.24–2.36	0.903	0.28–2.90
Electrocution	1.04	0.33–3.28	0.950	0.29–3.05
Animal bite injury	1.01	0.33–3.03	0.913	0.29–2.82
Injury by blunt object	0.63	0.22–1.80	0.779	0.26–2.28
Suffocation	1.45	0.08–26.26	1.373	0.07–25.63

Table 7. *Cont.*

Characteristics	Treatment Outcome (1 = Recovered/Improving; 0 = No Improvement)			
	Unadjusted		Adjusted	
	OR	95% CI	OR	95% CI
Age (in years)				
<10 years	Reference group		Reference group	
10–14 years	0.81	0.54–1.21	0.78	0.48–1.24
15–17 years	0.73	0.47–1.14	0.69	0.39–1.19
18–24 years	0.83	0.59–1.16	0.74	0.43–1.24
25–64 years	0.71 *	0.55–0.92	0.55 **	0.33–0.92
≥65 years	0.48 *	0.33–0.69	0.46 **	0.25–0.83
Sex				
Male	Reference group		Reference group	
Female	0.89	0.74–1.06	1.117285	0.87–1.42
Wealth quintile				
Lowest	Reference group		Reference group	
Low	1.00	0.77–1.29	1.06	0.80–1.38
Middle	1.07	0.83–1.38	1.15	0.88–1.50
High	0.86	0.66–1.11	0.95	0.72–1.24
Highest	0.89	0.68–1.16	1.10	0.82–1.46
District				
Chandpur/comilla	Reference group		Reference group	
Sirajganj	1.38 **	1.02–1.87	1.33	0.97–1.84
Sherpur	2.16 *	1.74–2.69	2.14	1.69–2.69
Narshingdi	2.14 *	1.69–2.71	2.03	1.58–2.59
Occupation				
Skilled labor (Professional)	Reference group		Reference group	
Agriculture	1.23	0.92–1.65	1.17	0.85–1.59
Business	0.97	0.68–1.37	0.96	0.67–1.37
Unskilled/domestic (Unskilled)	1.04	0.66–1.62	0.99	0.62–1.56
Rickshaw/bus (Transport worker)	1.32	0.87–2.01	1.29	0.83–1.99
Students	1.07	0.80–1.44	0.77	0.49–1.19
Retired/unemployed/housewife	0.71 **	0.55–0.93	0.72	0.52–1.00
Not applicable (children & others)	1.33	0.92–1.92	0.69	0.33–1.42
Education				
No education	Reference group		Reference group	
Primary	0.98	0.80–1.20	0.97	0.77–1.21
Secondary	0.92	0.74–1.14	0.96	0.73–1.23
A levels/college/Advanced/ Professional Degree	0.85	0.58–1.25	0.94	0.60–1.45
Not applicable (U5 children)	1.36	0.94–1.98	1.05	0.49–2.23

* $p < 0.01$, ** $p < 0.05$.

4. Discussion

Our study is one of the largest cross-sectional census in a developing country, covering more than 1 million people from different geographical areas in Bangladesh. About 8.7% of the surveyed population had at least one injury in the six months preceding the date of the interview. Overall, 81.7% of injury events received first aid from any provider, 79% of whom were not medically trained and 2.6% medically trained. Those who received first aid from a medically trained provider irrespective of age, sex, surgical intervention, occupation, SES, geographical location and education were 1.3 times more likely to recover or be in the process of improvement compared to those who did not receive first aid from trained providers.

We found that receiving first aid is quite common in rural areas of Bangladesh with over four-fifth of the events receiving first aid increasing as severity of injury increased. Our results suggest that first aid may be beneficial, and may reduce the severity of injuries, recovery time and improve survival. There may be other factors that influences the association of first aid and outcomes such as family support, transportation, cost of treatment and responses of health facility. Our results suggest first aid may play a role to reduce the severity of injuries and improves chances of survival [14]. Our study showed that first aid treatment from trained providers increased chances of recovery among severely injured individuals and hospitalized patients implying the importance of appropriate or correct first aid. Correct first aid treatment has been reported to reduce mortality by 1.8–4.5% for trauma events [23].

We found worse outcomes for patients who were housewives, as compared to skilled labor. This may be due to housewives being at greater risk of burn injuries, which are associated with worse prognosis. This underlines that outcome depends on type of injury [28,29]. Worse treatment outcomes were also found for those who obtained surgical treatment. This may be due to delays in obtaining surgery, already poor prognosis or postoperative surgical complications. We also found worse outcomes for older age groups. This may be due to falls which are common and devastating problems associated with identifiable risk factors like weakness, unsteady gait, confusion and medications [30]. Age has been identified as one of the most significant factors in determining outcomes after traumatic injuries and head injuries [31–33].

We found that the proportion who received first aid increased as injury severity increased. The more severe an injury was, the more people sought first aid from a medically trained provider. A review conducted on the recognition of childhood illness and care seeking behaviour in developing countries identified six studies all of which reported that if the caregiver perceived the child's illness as severe then they were more likely to seek care from trained providers [34]. Similar associations were found when severity of illness was defined by clinical criteria, such as rapid breathing, chest in-drawing [34].

In this study, largely untrained lay people present at the site of the event were the most common primary contacts that provided first aid to the injured. In addition, village doctors in rural Bangladesh are most commonly sought for medical care despite the existence of trained community based government and non-government health workers [35]. Multi-country evaluations of Integrated Management of Childhood Illness study showed that despite providing training for community based village health workers and availability of drugs in first level government facilities, care seeking for children under five years of age remained high from village doctors, with more than four-fifth receiving first aid treatment from an untrained provider [36]. Despite potential lack of relevant training of village doctors, when seeking medical care, the persistent use of them underlie an important consideration, when planning any intervention that seeks to improve first aid capacity through the availability of alternative trained health workers. These cultural preferences may negatively influence the acceptability and uptake of community-based first aid providers. Such potential intervention should consider cultural preference of service providers in order to maximize acceptability and uptake of interventions. Knowledge of first aid among lay people is often very limited and leads to harmful practices. A study to assess the knowledge of mothers on first aid for injuries to children arising from home accidents revealed that mothers answered an average of 11.0 (SD 5.3) out of 29 questions on first aid correctly [37]. In our study treatment outcome was not significantly different for those who received first aid from a non-medically trained provider, as compared with those who did not receive first aid and also demonstrated that those who received first aid from an untrained provider needed more time to recover reaffirming the importance of appropriateness of the first aid provided. Poor knowledge on appropriate first aid was also evident in studies conducted in developed countries [38]. A systematic review of first aid provided by lay people on trauma victims found that incorrect first aid was provided to 83.7% of cases [23]. Similarly, descriptive studies for common unintentional injuries such as burns, cuts, falls, suffocation among children in Turkey, South Africa, Ghana and Saudi-Arabia revealed that majority of the subjects had been treated with inappropriate interventions such as kitchen ingredients (yogurt, raw egg whites, honey, tomato paste) and household materials (toothpaste, aloe vera, Lavender oil) [39–42]. Although our study did not assess the appropriateness of the first aid, the negative findings associated with untrained providers raises questions on whether they provided appropriate first aid or not. A prior study from Bangladesh suggested that untrained providers mostly depend on secret spells and other 'spiritual' approaches with no physiological basis when providing first aid, and the custom is prevalent in both urban and rural areas [43].

Several studies indicate that training laypersons is beneficial and governments must have a more dynamic approach by promoting compulsory first aid education for example, in schools, when applying for a driving license, in the workplace and community with appropriate refresher courses [23,44–49]. In Bangladesh, CIPRB is implementing a community based first responder program in northern districts of Bangladesh [50]. The influence of SES on outcomes must also be considered during the implementation of community-based program. However, there is also need for rigorous studies to inform policy makers on the effectiveness of training on first aid.

In this census we found that the chances of recovery were significantly higher among patients in Sherpur districts compared to Chandpur/Comilla districts. This may be due availability of long-standing community-based injury intervention program, such as the first responder program by CIPRB, which created awareness [50].

Limitations

This study did not collect data on what procedures were applied as first aid and whether the procedures that were implemented as part of first aid provided were appropriate or not. Additionally, age, education, socioeconomic status, having paid employment, source of knowledge about first aid and having attended a training course on first aid have been reported as significant predictors of knowledge and practice among first aid providers [37–39]. However, such information was not collected within the scope of this study and provides potential for future research in establishing an association between first aid providers and injury outcomes.

5. Conclusions

This large population-based survey on injury in developing countries demonstrated that for non-fatal injury, untrained providers primarily provide first aid and surgical care. Public health interventions should be designed to develop the skills of the untrained providers as well as medically trained providers. Further, policies are needed to increase access to medically trained providers for the provision of first-aid for injuries. Such intervention needs to take into account cultural preferences for service providers in order to maximize acceptability and uptake of treatments.

Acknowledgments: This research was a part of the "Saving of children's Lives from Drowning (SOLID) in Bangladesh" project with funding support from Bloomberg Philanthropies. We would like to acknowledge the willingness and support provided by the respondents and their family members. We would also like to thank our all the data collectors and their supervisors for their hard work and ensuring quality data.

Author Contributions: Dewan Md Emdadul Hoque conceptualized the idea, conducted the analysis, wrote the first draft and managed subsequent revisions. Olakunle Alonge, Md Irteja Islam and Shumona Sharmin Salam conceptualized the idea, revised the analysis and edited the manuscript. Shumona Sharmin Salam, Irteja Islam and Qazi Sadeq-ur Rahman conducted analysis and worked on the subsequent revisions of the manuscript. Priyanka Agrawal, Aminur Rahman, Fazlur Rahman, Shams El-Arifeen and Adnan A. Hyder reviewed and edited the manuscript with critical insight.

Conflicts of Interest: The authors declare no conflict of interest. The funding sponsors had no role in the design of the study; in the collection, analyses, or interpretation of data; in the writing of the manuscript, and in the decision to publish the results.

Abbreviations

The following abbreviations are used in this manuscript:

LMICs	Low- and middle-income countries
OR	Odds ratio
CI	Confidence Interval
SOLID	Saving of children's Lives from Drowning
BHIS	Bangladesh Health and Injury Survey
IFRC	International Federation of Red Cross and Red Crescent Societies
SOLID	Saving of children's lives from drowning
CIPRB	Center for Injury Prevention and Research, Bangladesh

References

1. Gosselin, R.A.; Spiegel, D.A.; Coughlin, R.; Zirkle, L.G. Injuries: The neglected burden in developing countries. *Bull. World Health Org.* **2009**, *87*, 246. [CrossRef] [PubMed]
2. Jha, P.; Chaloupka, F.J.; Moore, J.; Gajalakshmi, V.; Gupta, P.C.; Peck, R.; Jamison, D.; Breman, J.; Measham, A.; Alleyne, G. Disease Control Priorities in Developing Countries 2006. Available online: http://citeseerx.ist.psu.edu/viewdoc/download?doi=10.1.1.668.8031&rep=rep1&type=pdf (accessed on 24 May 2017).
3. Stewart, K.-A.A.; Groen, R.S.; Kamara, T.B.; Farahzad, M.M.; Samai, M.; Cassidy, L.D.; Kushner, A.L.; Wren, S.M. Traumatic injuries in developing countries: Report from a nationwide cross-sectional survey of Sierra Leone. *JAMA Surg.* **2013**, *148*, 463–469. [CrossRef] [PubMed]
4. Murray, C.J.; Vos, T.; Lozano, R.; Naghavi, M.; Flaxman, A.D.; Michaud, C.; Ezzati, M.; Shibuya, K.; Salomon, J.A.; Abdalla, S. Disability-adjusted life years (DALYs) for 291 diseases and injuries in 21 regions, 1990–2010: A systematic analysis for the Global Burden of Disease Study 2010. *Lancet* **2013**, *380*, 2197–2223. [CrossRef]
5. Wang, H.D.; Naghavi, M.; Allen, C.; Barber, R.M.; Bhutta, Z.A.; Carter, A.; Casey, D.C.; Charlson, F.J.; Chen, A.Z.; Coates, M.M.; et al. Global, regional, and national life expectancy, all-cause mortality, and cause-specific mortality for 249 causes of death, 1980–2015: A systematic analysis for the Global Burden of Disease Study 2015. *Lancet* **2016**, *388*, 1459–1544. [CrossRef]
6. Vos, T.; Allen, C.; Arora, M.; Barber, R.M.; Bhutta, Z.A.; Brown, A.; Carter, A.; Casey, D.C.; Charlson, F.J.; Chen, A.Z. Global, regional, and national incidence, prevalence, and years lived with disability for 310 diseases and injuries, 1990–2015: A systematic analysis for the Global Burden of Disease Study 2015. *Lancet* **2016**, *388*, 1545–1602. [CrossRef]
7. Mahajan, N.; Aggarwal, M.; Raina, S.; Verma, L.R.; Mazta, S.R.; Gupta, B. Pattern of non-fatal injuries in road traffic crashes in a hilly area: A study from Shimla, North India. *Int. J. Crit. Illness Injury Sci.* **2013**, *3*, 190. [CrossRef] [PubMed]
8. Peltzer, K.; Phaswana-Mafuya, N.; Arokiasamy, P.; Biritwum, R.; Yawson, A.; Minicuci, N.; Williams, J.S.; Kowal, P.; Chatterji, S. Prevalence, circumstances and consequences of non-fatal road traffic injuries and other bodily injuries among older people in China, Ghana, India, Mexico, Russia and South Africa. *Afr. Saf. Promot.* **2015**, *13*, 59–77.
9. Molcho, M.; Harel, Y.; Pickett, W.; Scheidt, P.C.; Mazur, J.; Overpeck, M.D.; HBSC Violence and Injury Writing Group. The epidemiology of non-fatal injuries among 11-, 13- and 15-year old youth in 11 countries: Findings from the 1998 WHO-HBSC cross national survey. *Int. J. Injury Control Saf. Promot.* **2006**, *13*, 205–211. [CrossRef] [PubMed]
10. Lescohier, I.; Gallagher, S.S. Unintentional injury. In *Handbook of Adolescent Health Risk Behavior*; Springer: Berlin, Germany, 1996; pp. 225–258.
11. Rivara, F.P.; Grossman, D.C.; Cummings, P. Injury prevention. *N. Engl. J. Med.* **1997**, *337*, 543–548. [CrossRef] [PubMed]
12. Odero, W.; Garner, P.; Zwi, A. Road traffic injuries in developing countries: A comprehensive review of epidemiological studies. *Trop. Med. Int. Health* **1997**, *2*, 445–460. [CrossRef] [PubMed]

13. Birgul, P.; Ocaktan, M.E.; Akdur, R.; Soner, Y.M.; Sevil, I.; Safa, C. Evaluation of unintentional injuries sustained by children: A hospital based study from Ankara-Turkey. *Pak. J. Med. Sci.* **2013**, *29*, 832. [PubMed]
14. IFRC First Aid for a Safer Future: Updated Global Edition—Advocacy Report 2010. Available online: http://www.ifrc.org/PageFiles/53459/First%20aid%20for%20a%20safer%20future%20Updated%20global%20edition%20%20Advocacy%20report%202010%20(2).pdf?epslanguage=en (accessed on 24 May 2017).
15. Rahman, A.; Shafinaz, S.; Linnan, M. *Bangladesh Health and Injury Survey-Report on Children*; UNICEF: Dhaka, Bangladesh, 2005.
16. Giashuddin, S.M.; Rahman, A.; Rahman, F.; Mashreky, S.R.; Chowdhury, S.M.; Linnan, M.; Shafinaz, S. Socioeconomic inequality in child injury in Bangladesh—Implication for developing countries. *Int. J. Equity Health* **2009**, *8*, 7. [CrossRef] [PubMed]
17. Wood, F.M.; Phillips, M.; Jovic, T.; Cassidy, J.T.; Cameron, P.; Edgar, D.W. Water first aid is beneficial in humans post-burn: Evidence from a bi-national cohort study. *PLoS ONE* **2016**, *11*, e0147259. [CrossRef] [PubMed]
18. Larry, L.G.; Scheulen, J.J.; Munster, A.M. Chemical burns: Effect of prompt first aid. *J. Trauma Acute Care Surg.* **1982**, *22*, 420–423.
19. IFRC. *Law and First Aid: Promoting and Protecting Life-Saving Action*; International Federation of Red Cross and Red Crescent Societies: Geneva, Switzerland, 2015.
20. Shotland, R.L.; Heinold, W.D. Bystander response to arterial bleeding: Helping skills, the decision-making process, and differentiating the helping response. *J. Personal. Soc. Psychol.* **1985**, *49*, 347. [CrossRef]
21. Wei, Y.-L.; Chen, L.-L.; Li, T.-C.; Ma, W.-F.; Peng, N.-H.; Huang, L.-C. Self-efficacy of first aid for home accidents among parents with 0-to 4-year-old children at a metropolitan community health center in Taiwan. *Accid. Anal. Prev.* **2013**, *52*, 182–187. [CrossRef] [PubMed]
22. Arbon, P.; Hayes, J.; Woodman, R. First aid and harm minimization for victims of road trauma: A population study. *Prehosp. Disaster Med.* **2011**, *26*, 276–282. [CrossRef] [PubMed]
23. Tannvik, T.; Bakke, H.; Wisborg, T. A systematic literature review on first aid provided by laypeople to trauma victims. *Acta Anaesthesiol. Scand.* **2012**, *56*, 1222–1227. [CrossRef] [PubMed]
24. Sahu, S.A.; Agrawal, K.; Patel, P.K. Scald burn, a preventable injury: Analysis of 4306 patients from a major tertiary care center. *Burns* **2016**, *42*, 1844–1849. [CrossRef] [PubMed]
25. Hyder, A.A.; Alonge, O.; He, S.; Wadhwaniya, S.; Rahman, F.; Rahman, A.; Arifeen, S.E. Saving of Children's Lives from Drowning Project in Bangladesh. *Am. J. Prev. Med.* **2014**, *47*, 842–845. [CrossRef] [PubMed]
26. Hyder, A.A.; Alonge, O.; He, S.; Wadhwaniya, S.; Rahman, F.; Rahman, A.; Arifeen, S.E. A Framework for Addressing Implementation Gap in Global Drowning Prevention Interventions: Experiences from Bangladesh. *J. Health Popul. Nutr.* **2014**, *32*, 564–576. [PubMed]
27. Alonge, O.; Agrawal, P.; Talab, A.; Rahman, Q.A.; Rahman, F.; Arifeen, S.E.; Hyder, A.A. Fatal and Non-Fatal Injury Outcomes: Results from a Purposively Sampled Census of Seven Rural Sub-Districts in Bangladesh. *Lancet Glob. Health* **2017**, in press.
28. Edelman, L.S. Social and economic factors associated with the risk of burn injury. *Burns* **2007**, *33*, 958–965. [CrossRef] [PubMed]
29. Forjuoh, S.N. Burns in low-and middle-income countries: A review of available literature on descriptive epidemiology, risk factors, treatment, and prevention. *Burns* **2006**, *32*, 529–537. [CrossRef] [PubMed]
30. Rubenstein, L.Z. Falls in older people: Epidemiology, risk factors and strategies for prevention. *Age Ageing* **2006**, *35*, ii37–ii41. [CrossRef] [PubMed]
31. Demetriades, D.; Murray, J.; Martin, M.; Velmahos, G.; Salim, A.; Alo, K.; Rhee, P. Pedestrians injured by automobiles: Relationship of age to injury type and severity. *J. Am. Coll. Surg.* **2004**, *199*, 382–387. [CrossRef] [PubMed]
32. Luerssen, T.G.; Klauber, M.R.; Marshall, L.F. Outcome from head injury related to patient'age: A longitudinal prospective study of adult and pediatric head injury. *J. Neurosurg.* **1988**, *68*, 409–416. [CrossRef] [PubMed]
33. Disease Control Priorities Project. *Disease Control Priorities in Developing Countries*, 2nd ed.; Oxford University Press: New York, NY, USA, 2006; pp. 737–754.
34. Geldsetzer, P.; Williams, T.C.; Kirolos, A.; Mitchell, S.; Ratcliffe, L.A.; Kohli-Lynch, M.K.; Bischoff, E.J.L.; Cameron, S.; Campbell, H. The recognition of and care seeking behaviour for childhood illness in developing countries: A systematic review. *PLoS ONE* **2014**, *9*, e93427. [CrossRef] [PubMed]

35. Mahmood, S.S.; Iqbal, M.; Hanifi, S.; Wahed, T.; Bhuiya, A. Are "Village Doctors" in Bangladesh a curse or a blessing? *BMC Int. Health Hum. Rights* **2010**, *10*, 18. [CrossRef] [PubMed]

36. El Arifeen, S.; Blum, L.S.; Hoque, D.M.; Chowdhury, E.K.; Khan, R.; Black, R.E.; Victora, C.G.; Bryce, J. Integrated Management of Childhood Illness (IMCI) in Bangladesh: Early findings from a cluster-randomised study. *Lancet* **2004**, *364*, 1595–1602. [CrossRef]

37. Eldosoky, R.S. Home-related injuries among children: Knowledge, attitudes and practice about first aid among rural mothers. *East. Mediterr. Health J.* **2012**, *18*, 1021–1027. [PubMed]

38. Davies, M.; Maguire, S.; Okolie, C.; Watkins, W.; Kemp, A.M. How much do parents know about first aid for burns? *Burns* **2013**, *39*, 1083–1090. [CrossRef] [PubMed]

39. Alomar, M.; Rouqi, F.A.; Eldali, A. Knowledge, attitude, and belief regarding burn first aid among caregivers attending pediatric emergency medicine departments. *Burns* **2016**, *42*, 938–943. [CrossRef] [PubMed]

40. Karaoz, B. First-aid home treatment of burns among children and some implications at Milas, Turkey. *J. Emerg. Nurs.* **2010**, *36*, 111–114. [CrossRef] [PubMed]

41. Jonkheijm, A.; Zuidgeest, J.J.; van Dijk, M.; van As, A.B. Childhood unintentional injuries: Supervision and first aid provided. *Afr. J. Paediatr. Surg.* **2013**, *10*, 339–344. [CrossRef] [PubMed]

42. Gyedu, A.; Mock, C.; Nakua, E.; Otupiri, E.; Donkor, P.; Ebel, B.E. Pediatric First Aid Practices in Ghana: A Population-Based Survey. *World J. Surg.* **2015**, *39*, 1859–1866. [CrossRef] [PubMed]

43. Rahman, A. Bangladesh Health and Injury Survey: Report on Children. Available online: http://www.unicef.org/bangladesh/Bangladesh_Health_and_Injury_Survey-Report_on_Children.pdf (accessed on 24 May 2017).

44. Walsh, K.; Hili, S.; Dheansa, B. Compulsory teaching of first aid in UK schools—A missed opportunity? *Burns* **2016**, *42*, 946–947. [CrossRef] [PubMed]

45. Reveruzzi, B.; Buckley, L.; Sheehan, M. School-Based First Aid Training Programs: A Systematic Review. *J. Sch. Health* **2016**, *86*, 266–272. [CrossRef] [PubMed]

46. Olumide, A.O.; Asuzu, M.C.; Kale, O.O. Effect of First Aid Education on First Aid Knowledge and Skills of Commercial Drivers in South West Nigeria. *Prehosp. Disaster Med.* **2015**, *30*, 579–585. [CrossRef] [PubMed]

47. VanderBurgh, D.; Jamieson, R.; Beardy, J.; Ritchie, S.D.; Orkin, A. Community-based first aid: A program report on the intersection of community-based participatory research and first aid education in a remote Canadian Aboriginal community. *Rural Remote Health* **2014**, *14*, 2537. [PubMed]

48. Vakili, M.A.; Mohjervatan, A.; Heydari, S.T.; Akbarzadeh, A.; Hosini, N.S.; Alizad, F.; Arasteh, P.; Moghasemi, M.J. The efficacy of a first aid training course for drivers: An experience from northern Iran. *Chin. J. Traumatol.* **2014**, *17*, 289–292. [PubMed]

49. Oliver, E.; Cooper, J.; McKinney, D. Can first aid training encourage individuals' propensity to act in an emergency situation? A pilot study. *Emerg. Med. J.* **2014**, *31*, 518–520. [CrossRef] [PubMed]

50. Rahman, A.; Mecrow, T.S.; Mashreky, S.R.; Rahman, A.K.; Nusrat, N.; Khanam, M.; Scarr, J.; Linnan, M. Feasibility of a first responder programme in rural Bangladesh. *Resuscitation* **2014**, *85*, 1088–1092. [CrossRef] [PubMed]

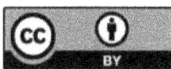

International Journal of
*Environmental Research
and Public Health*

MDPI

Article

Caregiver Supervision Practices and Risk of Childhood Unintentional Injury Mortality in Bangladesh

Khaula Khatlani [1,2], Olakunle Alonge [1,*], Aminur Rahman [3], Dewan Md. Emdadul Hoque [4], Al-Amin Bhuiyan [3], Priyanka Agrawal [1] and Fazlur Rahman [3]

[1]   Johns Hopkins International Injury Research Unit, Department of International Health, Johns Hopkins Bloomberg School of Public Health, Baltimore, MD 21205, USA; khaulakhatlani@gmail.com (K.K.); pagrawa6@jhu.edu (P.A.)
[2]   Department of Preventive Medicine, Griffin Hospital, Derby, CT 06418, USA
[3]   Centre for Injury Prevention and Research, Bangladesh (CIPRB), Dhaka 1206, Bangladesh; aminur@ciprb.org (A.R.); al_amin_prime@yahoo.com (A.-A.B.); fazlur@ciprb.org (F.R.)
[4]   International Centre for Diarrheal Diseases Research in Bangladesh (ICDDR,B), Dhaka 1212, Bangladesh; emdad@icddrb.org
*   Correspondence: oalonge1@jhu.edu; Tel.: +1-410-502-3946

Academic Editor: David C. Schwebel
Received: 15 February 2017; Accepted: 5 May 2017; Published: 11 May 2017

Abstract: Unintentional injury-related mortality rate, including drowning among children under five, is disproportionately higher in low- and middle-income countries. The evidence links lapse of supervision with childhood unintentional injury deaths. We determined the relationship between caregiver supervision and unintentional injury mortality among children under five in rural Bangladesh. We conducted a nested, matched, case-control study within the cohort of a large-scale drowning prevention project in Bangladesh, "SOLID—Saving of Children's Lives from Drowning". From the baseline survey of the project, 126 cases (children under five with unintentional injury deaths) and 378 controls (alive children under five) were selected at case-control ratio of 1:3 and individually matched on neighborhood. The association between adult caregiver supervision and fatal injuries among children under five was determined in a multivariable conditional logistic regression analysis, and reported as adjusted matched odds ratio (MOR) with 95% confidence intervals (CIs). Children under five experiencing death due to unintentional injuries, including drowning, had 3.3 times increased odds of being unsupervised as compared with alive children (MOR = 3.3, 95% CI: 1.6–7.0), while adjusting for children's sex, age, socioeconomic index, and adult caregivers' age, education, occupation, and marital status. These findings are concerning and call for concerted, multi-sectoral efforts to design community-level prevention strategies. Public awareness and promotion of appropriate adult supervision strategies are needed.

Keywords: childhood unintentional injuries; drowning; drowning mortality; caregiver supervision; children under five; developing country; Bangladesh

1. Introduction

Unintentional injuries among children are a major public health concern and a cause of substantial childhood morbidity and mortality [1]. The leading mechanisms of unintentional injuries among children less than 15 years are drowning, road traffic injuries, burns, and falls [2]. Among children aged 5 years and below, drowning is the leading cause of injury death globally, and over 90% of these deaths occur in low- and middle-income countries (LMICs) [3,4]. In Bangladesh, drowning accounts for 43% of all deaths in children aged 1–4 years. A child drowns every 30 min in Bangladesh, and 80% of these deaths occur within or around the home environment [3–5].

Whereas multiple factors contribute to the occurrence of an injury event among children under five years of age, lack of appropriate supervision is, however, considered to be a major contributing factor [6]. Supervision, in general, could be summarized by domains of attentiveness, proximity, and continuity, and can be considered as "the interaction of attentional behaviors and physical proximity extended in time" [1,6]. There is neither a consensus on the definition of supervision in the literature, nor on the quality of supervision required for preventing childhood unintentional injuries [7]. Indeed, distinctive environmental and behavioral factors shape parental attributes and parenting styles affecting the quality of supervision and occurrence of childhood unintentional injuries [8,9]. The lack of a standardized validated instrument tailored especially to the sociocultural contexts in LMICs further makes it difficult to explore supervision [6].

The evidence linking lapse of adult supervision with childhood unintentional injury deaths is mainly based on descriptive data from high-income countries (HICs), and few if any have assessed this relationship in a LMIC setting [10–19]. Hence, the objective of our study is to determine the relationship between adult caregiver supervision and unintentional injury deaths among children aged five years and below in rural Bangladesh. We hope that our study will contribute to the understanding of the role of supervision in preventing childhood unintentional injuries in LMICs, and to the design of effective childhood injury prevention strategies.

2. Materials and Methods

2.1. Study Design, Setting and Participants

We conducted a matched case-control study nested within the "SOLID—Saving of Children's Lives from Drowning" project, which is a large-scale drowning prevention project in Bangladesh [20]. One of the aims of the SOLID project was to describe the burden and risk factors of drowning, and other injuries, among young children in Bangladesh. The SOLID project included a baseline census conducted in 51 unions (out of 83 unions) from seven sub-districts of rural Bangladesh: Matlab North, Matlab South, Daudkandi, Chandpur Sadar, Raiganj, Sherpur Sadar, and Manohardi. The census collected sociodemographic and injury outcome data on approximately 1.2 million people from 270,387 households.

The cases selected for our matched case-control study were children under five (male and female) that died from unintentional injuries in the SOLID census area, and the controls were similarly aged children who were alive over the same period. To ensure homogeneity of household, environmental, and socioeconomic characteristics between cases and controls, we selected controls from a neighborhood as close to their respective cases as possible. Controls were selected from the same Bari but a different household as that of the cases. A Bari is a collection of 2–10 households living in close proximity and within the same geographical compound; these households share resources including housing, water, food, and space for animals. If no suitable controls were found from a different household within the same Bari as a case, then the controls were selected from the same Bari and the same household or from an adjacent Bari within the same village.

Three controls were selected for every case to yield a matching ratio of 3:1. Our case-control study included all 126 cases of children under five who died due to unintentional injuries in the last 12 months prior to the census. In all, the sample size for our matched case-control study was 504 (126 cases and 378 controls). This sample size has more than 90% power to detect an odds ratio of 2 in mortality due to unintentional injuries, comparing cases to control, and assuming that the prevalence of supervision is 50% in the general population.

2.2. Study Variables and Study Tool

Unintentional injury was operationally defined as any household member who sought treatment or lost at least one working day or could not go to the school for at least one day due to an injury event [20]. The injury events listed included suicide, transport injury, violence, fall, cut injury, burn, drowning, poisoning, machine injury, electrocution, animal bite injury, injury by blunt object, suffocation, and others. We further categorized all injuries based on intent, and described them as: unintentional injuries, self-harm, and violence [21]. Drowning was defined as "the process of experiencing respiratory impairment from submersion/immersion in liquid" [22].

Death from unintentional injuries was the main outcome variable, and this data was collected over a one-year recall period. Supervision was the main exposure variable. Since physical proximity between a child and an adult caregiver is most closely correlated with supervision, we used physical proximity as a proxy indicator for supervision in our study [1,23]. Based on prior injury literature in children, a child was considered in proximity of the adult caregiver if both the child and the adult caregiver were at the same location, either inside or outside of the home during the review period [24,25]. We described specific locations inside and outside of a typical home in rural Bangladesh such that the co-location of both the child and adult caregiver at the same location would put the adult caregiver at arm's length of the child. To avoid any social desirability bias, we divided a day into different periods and independently assessed the specific location of the child and adult caregiver at each of those periods. In this study, we only considered supervision during a review period between 9 am and 1 pm, as the majority of unintentional injury deaths (mainly drowning) in Bangladesh are reported to take place during this time period [5].

We defined an adult caregiver as the head of household or any adult 18 years of age or older who had primary responsibility for overseeing the child's welfare during the period under review. While we recognized that older children at times could "supervise" younger children, the injury literature suggests that supervision by an adult may be more effective compared to supervision by an older child (especially an older child below 13 years of age) [26]. Supervision conducted by children younger than 13 years could in fact increase injury risk for the child that is being supervised [26].

We obtained all information using questionnaires designed based on guidelines for injury surveillance by the World Health Organization (WHO) [27]. The questionnaires were used to collect data on injury mortality and morbidity, sociodemographic characteristics, environmental factors, supervision practices, and drowning related factors and prevention practices for households with children under five [3,20].

2.3. Data Collection Procedure

Two sets of trained data collectors administered the questionnaires. Data were obtained from either the head of the household or any adult 18 years and older who was present in the house during face-to-face interviews. The first set of data collectors gathered information on household characteristics, birth history, household environment, and death confirmation. If an injury was reported, the second set of data collectors visited the household to collect data on injury morbidity, injury mortality, and mechanism of injury. The data collectors were adults 18 years and older who had completed at least secondary school education, and had undergone 15 days of field training. The field training included modules on the questionnaires, operational manual, survey implementation, research ethics, and data management. An initial pilot-testing of the questionnaires revealed a high percentage of agreement (>80%) regarding the data collected from the same households by different data collectors. The activities of the data collectors were supervised by the field supervisors, who reported directly to a field research or sub-district manager, and the managers reported directly to the central office. Daily collation of data was done at the union level with oversight from the field supervisor, after which data were transmitted to the sub-district level for preliminary cleaning before transmission to the central office. All questionnaires were translated from English to Bangla (Bangladesh's local language), and were back-translated and pre-tested in the field. Ethical clearance was obtained from the Institutional Review Boards at Johns Hopkins Bloomberg School of Public Health (JHSPH), International Centre for Diarrheal Disease Research, Bangladesh (ICDDR,B) and Centre for Injury Prevention Research Bangladesh (CIPRB) (Ethical Approval Code 00004746). The study was conducted in accordance with the Declaration of Helsinki.

2.4. Statistical Analysis

First, we obtained data on adult caregivers' sociodemographic characteristics for the selected cases and controls and linked these with the supervision and injury mortality data from the SoLiD baseline census. Second, we described the frequencies and percentages of all included variables. Third, we computed the unadjusted matched odds ratio (MOR) of unintentional injury deaths among children under five with 95% confidence intervals (CIs) using simple conditional logistic regression. Fourth, we described a multivariable model for the odds of unintentional injury deaths among children under five with adult caregiver supervision as the main explanatory variable, using a multiple conditional logistic regression. We added other predictors to the multivariate model, one at a time, checking the model significance each time based on the likelihood ratio test ($p < 0.05$). Last, we reported the adjusted MOR with 95% CI for adult caregiver supervision and other predictors from the multivariate model.

To see if the odds ratios in our study approached the relative risk, we tested the rare disease assumption by assessing the prevalence of unintentional injury-related mortality among children under five from our source population. The characteristics of the selected controls and all living children under five from our source population were also compared to check if the controls were truly representative of our source population. We conducted all statistical analyses using STATA version 14 (StataCorp. 2015. Stata Statistical Software: Release 14. StataCorp LP, College Station, TX, USA).

3. Results

The SOLID baseline census database had a total of 112,664 children under five; 126 injury deaths were reported among these children over a one-year recall period. All injury deaths were unintentional except for one case that was undetermined. All unintentional injury deaths resulted from drowning except for 14 (11%) cases. Of the 14 cases, 5 (4%) were road traffic injuries, 4 (3.2%) suffocation, 2 (1.6%) cut injury, and 1 (0.8%) death each due to unintentional poisoning and animal bite injury. Three hundred seventy-eight (378) controls were selected at a 1:3 case-control ratio and matched on geographical location/neighborhood.

3.1. Baseline Characteristics of Children under Five and Their Caregivers

Overall, 18.4% of children were supervised (cases 8.7%; control 21.7%) (Tables 1 and 2). A higher proportion of cases were males (cases 53.2%; controls 48.7%), and in the 1–4 years age group (cases 94.4%; controls 81.2%) (Table 2). The minimum age of the adult caregivers in our study was 18 years; overall 83.3% of the adult caregivers were in the age category 25–64 years (Table 3). Only 4.6% of children in the study had adult caregivers with education beyond secondary level (cases 3.2%; controls 5%). In Bangladesh, grades 1–5 are considered primary education, grades 6–12 secondary, and advanced level is grades 13 and above. The most common occupation among adult caregivers was agriculture/farming (28.6%), followed by those who were retired/unemployed/housewives (21%). A greater percentage of adult caregivers of cases were older than 65 years (cases 20.6%; controls 10.6%) and were transport workers (cases 11.1%; controls 6.1%). On the other hand, more adult caregivers of controls were traders as compared to cases (cases 13.5%; controls 20.6%) (Table 3). Both the cases and the controls were similar in terms of socioeconomic index as well as adult caregivers' education and marital status.

Table 1. Baseline characteristics of children under five in the entire population.

Characteristics	Total (n = 112,664) n (%)	Injury Death (n = 126) n (%)	Alive (n = 112,538) n (%)	p-Value
Supervision:				<0.01
Yes	20,569 (18.3)	11 (8.7)	20,558 (18.3)	
No	92,095 (81.7)	115 (91.3)	91,980 (81.7)	
Sex:				0.6
Female	55,372 (49.1)	59 (46.8)	55,313 (49.2)	
Male	57,292 (50.9)	67 (53.2)	57,225 (50.8)	
Age (years):				<0.01
<1	22,141 (19.7)	7 (5.6)	22,134 (19.7)	
1–4	90,523 (80.3)	119 (94.4)	90,404 (80.3)	
Socioeconomic index:				0.9
Lowest	22,946 (20.4)	26 (20.6)	22,920 (20.4)	
Low	20,355 (18.0)	26 (20.6)	20,329 (18.0)	
Middle	22,413 (19.9)	24 (19.1)	22,389 (19.9)	
High	22,270 (19.8)	23 (18.3)	22,247 (19.8)	
Highest	24,680 (21.9)	27 (21.4)	24,653 (21.9)	

Table 2. Characteristics of children under five, cases and selected controls.

Characteristics	Total (n = 504) n (%)	Cases (n = 126) n (%)	Controls (n = 378) n (%)	Unadjusted MOR (95% CI)
Supervision:				
Yes	93 (18.4)	11 (8.7)	82 (21.7)	1.0
No	411 (81.6)	115 (91.3)	296 (78.3)	2.9 (1.5–5.7)
Sex:				
Female	253 (50.2)	59 (46.8)	194 (51.3)	1.0
Male	251 (49.8)	67 (53.2)	184 (48.7)	1.2 (0.8–1.8)
Age (years):				
<1	78 (15.5)	7 (5.6)	71 (18.8)	1.0
1–4	426 (84.5)	119 (94.4)	307 (81.2)	3.8 (1.7–8.5)
Socioeconomic index:				
Lowest	102 (20.2)	26 (20.6)	76 (20.1)	1.2 (0.6–2.3)
Low	105 (20.8)	26 (20.6)	79 (20.9)	1.1 (0.6–2.1)
Middle	106 (21.0)	24 (19.1)	82 (21.7)	1.0
High	98 (19.4)	23 (18.3)	75 (19.8)	1.05 (0.5–2.1)
Highest	93 (18.6)	27 (21.4)	66 (17.5)	1.5 (0.7–3.1)

Table 3. Characteristics of adult caregivers of selected cases and controls.

Characteristics	Total (n = 504) n (%)	Cases (n = 126) n (%)	Controls (n = 378) n (%)	Unadjusted MOR (95% CI)
Age (years):				
18–24	18 (3.6)	2 (1.6)	16 (4.2)	0.4 (0.1–1.7)
25–64	420 (83.3)	98 (77.8)	322 (85.2)	1.0
≥65	66 (13.1)	26 (20.6)	40 (10.6)	2.7 (1.4–5.1)
Education:				
None	181 (35.9)	49 (38.9)	132 (34.9)	1.0
Primary	179 (35.5)	49 (38.9)	130 (34.4)	0.9 (0.6–1.6)
Secondary	121 (24.0)	24 (19.0)	97 (25.7)	0.6 (0.3–1.3)
Advanced level and above	23 (4.6)	4 (3.2)	19 (5.0)	0.5 (0.1–1.6)
Occupation *:				
Trading	95 (18.9)	17 (13.5)	78 (20.6)	1.0
Agriculture/farming	144 (28.6)	35 (27.8)	109 (28.8)	1.5 (0.7–2.9)
Skilled labor	94 (18.7)	25 (19.8)	69 (18.3)	1.7 (0.8–3.4)
Unskilled labor	25 (5.0)	6 (4.8)	19 (5.0)	1.4 (0.4–4.3)
Transport worker	37 (7.3)	14 (11.1)	23 (6.1)	3.0 (1.2–7.2)
Student	2 (0.4)	1 (0.8)	1 (0.3)	4.4 (0.3–73.7)
Retired/Unemployed/Housewife	106 (21.0)	28 (22.2)	78 (20.6)	1.6 (0.8–3.4)
Marital status:				
Married	476 (94.4)	120 (95.2)	356 (94.2)	1.0
Never married/divorced/widowed	28 (5.6)	6 (4.8)	22 (5.8)	0.8 (0.3–2.1)

* Information on the caregivers' occupation was missing for one control (total missing n = 1 (0.2%); control missing n = 1 (0.3%)).

3.2. Univariate and Multivariable Analysis

Based on the univariate model, supervision (unsupervised child compared to supervised), child's age (1–4 years compared to those <1 year), adult caregiver's age (≥65 years compared to those 24–65 years), and adult caregiver's occupation (transport workers compared to traders) were significantly associated with unintentional injury-related mortality among children under five (Table 4). Based on the final multivariable model, children under five who died from unintentional injuries had 3.3 times increased odds of being unsupervised as compared to alive children (MOR = 3.3, 95% CI: 1.6–7.0), while adjusting for children's sex (male, female), age (<1, 1–4 years), socioeconomic index (lowest, low, middle, high, highest), and adult caregivers' age (18–24, 25–64, ≥65 years), education (none, secondary, A levels and above), occupation (trading, agriculture, skilled labor, unskilled labor, transport worker, student, retired/unemployed/housewife), and marital status (married, never married/divorced/widowed) (Table 4). In the adjusted analysis, likelihood of dying due to unintentional injuries also increased significantly if the child was aged 1–4 years as opposed to less than 1 year of age (OR = 5.2, 95% CI: 2.2–12.2), had an adult caregiver aged 65 years and above compared to age 25–64 years, (OR = 3.4, 95% CI: 1.5–7.6), and whose adult caregiver was a transport worker compared to a trader (OR = 3.4, 95% CI: 1.3–9.0). A child's sex and socioeconomic status, and adult caregiver's education and marital status were not significantly associated with unintentional injury-related mortality (Table 4).

Table 4. Association of unintentional injury-related mortality with adult caregiver supervision and other independent variables.

Characteristics	Unadjusted MOR (95% CI)	Adjusted MOR (95% CI)
Supervision:		
Yes	1.0	1.0
No	2.9 (1.5–5.7)	3.3 (1.6–7.0)
Sex of the child:		
Female	1.0	1.0
Male	1.2 (0.8–1.8)	1.1 (0.7–1.8)
Age of the child (years):		
<1	1.0	1.0
1–4	3.8 (1.7–8.5)	5.2 (2.2–12.2)
Socioeconomic index:		
Lowest	1.2 (0.6–2.3)	0.7 (0.3–1.5)
Low	1.1 (0.6–2.1)	0.8 (0.4–1.7)
Middle	1.0	1.0
High	1.05 (0.5–2.1)	0.8 (0.4–1.7)
Highest	1.5 (0.7–3.1)	1.2 (0.5–2.6)
Caregiver's age (years):		
18–24	0.4 (0.1–1.7)	0.3 (0.03–2.2)
25–64	1.0	1.0
≥65	2.7 (1.4–5.1)	3.4 (1.5–7.6)
Caregiver's education:		
None	1.0	1.0
Primary	0.9 (0.6–1.6)	0.9 (0.5–1.6)
Secondary	0.6 (0.3–1.3)	0.7 (0.3–1.4)
A levels and above	0.5 (0.1–1.6)	0.4 (0.1–1.5)
Caregiver's occupation:		
Trading	1.0	1.0
Agriculture/farming	1.5 (0.7–2.9)	1.4 (0.6–3.0)
Skilled labor	1.7 (0.8–3.4)	2.0 (0.9–4.3)
Unskilled labor	1.4 (0.4–4.3)	1.9 (0.6–6.4)
Transport worker	3.0 (1.2–7.2)	3.4 (1.3–9.0)
Student	4.4 (0.3–73.7)	-
Retired/Unemployed/Housewife	1.6 (0.8–3.4)	1.4 (0.6–3.3)
Caregiver's marital status:		
Married	1.0	1.0
Never married/divorced/widowed	0.8 (0.3–2.1)	0.4 (0.1–1.4)

3.3. Comparison of Controls with the Source Population

The prevalence of unintentional injury was very low in our source data—126 per 112,664 total population or 0.1%. A comparison of the controls with other children under five from our source data did not yield any significant difference with respect to supervision status, age, sex, and socioeconomic status (Tables S1 and S2). Hence, we concluded that the rare disease assumption is reasonable given our data.

4. Discussion

To our knowledge, our study is the first epidemiological study to have explicitly explored the relationship between adult supervision and unintentional injury deaths among children under five years of age in a rural setting of a developing country. We highlighted the protective role of adult supervision on fatal unintentional injuries of young children, especially drowning in rural Bangladesh. Our study suggested that the risk of unintentional injury mortality (mainly drowning) was three times higher among children younger than five years when they were not in close proximity of an adult caregiver, adjusting for covariates.

As far as the protective role of adult supervision in childhood unintentional injury prevention in an aquatic environment is concerned, our findings validate earlier studies [10,11,15,16,18,19,23,28,29]. While our findings are alarming, they are of public health significance. Once drowning occurs in a young child, death is almost certain and rapid. Even in instances where a child receives timely and adequate cardiopulmonary resuscitation, that child could still be faced with substantial morbidity such as neurological impairment [16]. Rural Bangladesh is mainly an agrarian society in which people build homes in close proximity to water bodies to have easy access to water for farming, bathing, cleaning, washing clothes/dishes, and recreational activities [5]. While our study highlights drowning as a main external cause of unintentional injury death among children under five (and the contribution of lack of supervision given Bangladeshi setting), lack of supervision is able to contribute to other leading external causes of injury in other settings depending on the environmental factors in those settings.

Even though safety barriers between residences and water bodies can be an effective environmental intervention for drowning, it is nearly impossible to fence large natural water bodies, as in the case of Bangladesh [30–32]. Young children can experience drowning due to lapses in adult supervision despite physical barriers between the children and the water bodies [10,16]. Moreover, children under five who have the highest risk of dying due to drowning are seldom proficient swimmers [33,34]. The notion that giving swimming lessons to young children could reduce drowning deaths lacks sufficient evidence; in fact, there is recommendation against this strategy for children less than two years of age [31]. Therefore, primary prevention in the form of adequate adult supervision cannot be overemphasized in preventing childhood drowning deaths [23,31,32].

While the importance of attentiveness and continuity—two other pillars of the hierarchical model of supervision—cannot be overlooked, our results suggest that proximity could be used as a reasonable indicator of supervision in a resource-poor setting [6]. Physical proximity of the adult caregiver is regarded as the most vital component of supervision because it significantly diminishes risk-taking behavior among children [1,23,35]. This is crucial, as the assessment of supervision is most often difficult and subjective, especially in the absence of a standard tool. Morrengiello and House designed the Parents Supervision Attributes Profile Questionnaire in order to measure parental attributes which could indirectly predict parental supervision behavior and subsequent child risk-taking behavior [35]. However, it is not yet determined if the questionnaire is applicable in other sociocultural environments with different structural factors or in LMIC settings. It is noteworthy that the sociocultural environment of a community influences parental perceptions and cognitive behavior, which in turn affects the kind and level of supervision deemed appropriate for children [7]. The sociocultural differences that predispose children to greater injury risks have, however, not been established in the literature. To this end, future studies to develop supervision tools adapted for various settings and to examine the relationship between sociocultural differences in supervision and child injury risk would be desirable.

Our results indicate that children aged 1–4 years are at significantly higher risk of unintentional injury mortality (mostly drowning), which is consistent with other studies [5,11]. Children aged 1–4 years are mobile, and they exhibit a higher risk-taking behavior than infants; thus, they are more exposed to the risk of unintentional injuries and require closer supervision [16]. As children get older, parents tend to underrate close supervision or misperceive children as efficient enough to deal with the injury risk themselves [36]. Current guidelines for child injury prevention should be explicit on the need to educate adult caregivers about providing continuous supervision to young children in hazardous environments [34,36]. Injury prevention programs, including drowning prevention programs, need to educate adult caregivers about children's lack of motor skills required for self-rescue in event of an injury or near-submersion [11,36]. An adult caregiver's knowledge of the child's development has been shown to influence quality of supervision [37].

The finding of adult caregivers 65 years of age and older as a significant risk factor for childhood unintentional injury mortality is unique. Potential mechanisms could be elderly caregivers being limited physically to keep a close eye on the children, or intervene in the event of submersion in water. Moreover, elderly caregivers, such as grandparents, face considerable stress, exhaustion, and poor physical health and mental health conditions, which may impair them in being able to provide adequate or continuous supervision to young children [38–40]. Scarce data have, however, examined the role of supervision by elderly caregivers and child unintentional injury mortality, and the mechanisms through which more or less frequent injuries may occur under such observation. A study suggested protective, though statistically insignificant effect of grandparents' supervision on medically-attended childhood injuries [41]. In contrast, our study focused on unintentional injury deaths, the majority of which were due to drowning, requiring caregivers to be physically active, vigilant, and close enough to young children to intervene and prevent such an incident from happening. However, adult caregivers above 65 years may not be able to do so due to their functional limitations. This calls for the promotion of low-cost and community-based programs that support child supervision by trained adults in LMICs, such as crèches (day care centers) [42]. Such programs have been demonstrated to reduce drowning and other unintentional injuries among children through the provision of close adult supervision in a safe environment [42]. The crèches allow working adults to perform their jobs, while similarly aged adults (crèche mothers) supervise children.

As expected, male children were more likely to die from unintentional injuries than females [5,10,11]. Male children demonstrate higher risk-taking behavior while parents tend to supervise female children more closely [25,43]. It should be noted that unintentional injuries among children are a complex interplay of a child's characteristics, environmental factors, parental beliefs, and supervision practices [25]. Consistent with prior studies, our study suggests that the risk of unintentional injury-related mortality decreased linearly with increasing level of adult caregiver's education, though the results were not statistically significant [5]. Our finding of a significantly increased risk of child unintentional injury death among children supervised by adult caregivers who are transport workers compared with traders is remarkable and worthy of further inquiry, especially given that this association is independent of socioeconomic status. It would be interesting to explore if fatal injury events among children occurred at the same time and place where adult caregivers performed their jobs as transport workers. This information would be especially critical, in terms of childhood drowning and adult caregivers involved in water transport; however, lack of data prevented us from evaluating this further in our current study.

Our study is the first large population-based study in a LMIC to assess contribution of lack of adult supervision towards unintentional injury-related deaths among children under five. Using the rare disease assumption, our odds ratios could be used as a good approximation of relative risk, further strengthening the evidence we present in this study. We addressed selection bias by using a nested matched case-control study design and by demonstrating through analysis that the controls were truly representative of the source population [44] (Tables S1 and S2).

Our study is not without limitations. First, we did not assess other domains of supervision— attentiveness and continuity—in this study due to lack of data. Based on prior evidence, we used physical proximity of the child with the adult caregiver as a proxy and assumed that having a young child within an adult caregiver's reach enabled the adult caregiver to watch/listen to the child (attentiveness) without considerable interruption (continuity) [23]. Second, the cut-off age of 18 years that we had used for defining an adult caregiver may have excluded appropriate supervision by older children (especially those older than 13 years). We, however, explored this and did not find that the cut-off age differentially affected the cases compared to the controls. Hence, we maintained our conclusion about the relationship between adult supervision and child unintentional injury deaths. However, our study findings may not be generalizable to populations where supervision is provided mainly by older children or by multiple caregivers.

Third, we also did not include all of the alive children under five population as the comparator, but we did demonstrate that the selected controls were a true representation of the source population. Fourth, our model omits other important predictors of childhood unintentional injury such as, household size, adult caregivers' substance abuse, beliefs, and personality, and children's attributes including risk taking behavior and temperament due to lack of data. Fifth, to avoid losing power, we did not conduct sensitivity analysis based on the child's age to account for the differences in supervision practices with respect to mobility of children. However, as the issue equally affects both cases and controls, we can maintain our conclusion about the relationship between adult supervision and child unintentional injury deaths. Last, it should be noted that the most common cause of unintentional injury mortality could be different if the study were to be replicated in another developing country, with an entirely different landscape than Bangladesh [45].

Our study is generalizable to other rural LMIC settings with a profile similar to rural Bangladesh. We advocate for approaches for enhancing adequate adult supervision of young children to decrease child injury risks, including drowning, in LMICs.

5. Conclusions

Children under five years of age who died from unintentional injury-related deaths had a 3-fold higher likelihood of being unsupervised by an adult as compared to similarly aged living children, after matching for neighborhood factors and adjusting for children's sex, age, socioeconomic status, and adult caregivers' age, education, occupation, and marital status. Children's age, and adult caregiver's age and occupation were other significant predictors of deaths from unintentional injuries among these children. These findings are concerning and call for concerted, multi-sectoral efforts to deliver effective community-level prevention strategies. Public awareness and promotion of appropriate adult supervision strategies are needed to progress toward this goal.

Supplementary Materials: The following are available online at www.mdpi.com/1660-4601/14/5/515/s1, Table S1: Comparison of proportions of independent variables between controls and alive children under five years of age in the source population, Table S2: Comparison of proportions of independent variables between controls and total children under five years age in the source population.

Acknowledgments: We would like to acknowledge Samantha Hauf and Eileen O'Brien for their editorial support in finalizing the manuscript.

Author Contributions: Olakunle Alonge conceived the paper; Olakunle Alonge and Khaula Khatlani performed the statistical analysis; Khaula Khatlani, Olakunle Alonge, Aminur Rahman, Dewan Md. Emdadul Hoque, Al-Amin Bhuiyan, Priyanka Agrawal, and Fazlur Rahman interpreted the results; Khaula Khatlani drafted the initial manuscript; Olakunle Alonge, Aminur Rahman, Dewan Md. Emdadul Hoque, Al-Amin Bhuiyan, Priyanka Agrawal, and Fazlur Rahman provided feedback on the content of the manuscript and editorial support. Khaula Khatlani and Olakunle Alonge modified subsequent drafts. All authors read and approved the final draft of the manuscript.

Conflicts of Interest: The authors declare no conflict of interest.

Abbreviations

The following abbreviations are used in this manuscript:

CIPRB	The Center for Injury Prevention Research Bangladesh
95% CI	95% confidence interval
HICs	high income countries
ICDDR,B	International Center for Diarrheal Disease Research, Bangladesh
LMICs	Low- and middle-income countries
MOR	matched odds ratio
SOLID	Saving of Children's Lives from Drowning

References

1. Morrongiello, B.A. Caregiver supervision and child-injury risk: I. Issues in defining and measuring supervision; II. Findings and directions for future research. *J. Pediatr. Psychol.* **2005**, *30*, 536–552. [CrossRef] [PubMed]
2. World Healt Organization. Global Health Estimates 2014: Causes of Death by Age, Sex and Region, 2000–2012. Available online: http://www.who.int/healthinfo/global_burden_disease/en/ (accessed on 12 September 2016).

3. Hyder, A.A.; Alonge, O.; He, S.; Wadhwaniya, S.; Rahman, F.; El Arifeen, S. A framework for addressing implementation gap in global drowning prevention interventions: Experiences from Bangladesh. *J. Health Popul. Nutr.* **2014**, *32*, 564–576. [PubMed]
4. World Health Organization. WHO Global Report on Drowning: Preventing A Leading Killer. 2014. Available online: http://apps.who.int/iris/bitstream/10665/143893/1/9789241564786_eng.pdf?ua=1&ua= (accessed on 20 December 2014).
5. Hossain, M.; Mani, K.K.; Sidik, S.M.; Hayati, K.S.; Rahman, A.K. Socio-demographic, environmental and caring risk factors for childhood drowning deaths in Bangladesh. *BMC Pediatr.* **2015**, *15*, 114. [CrossRef] [PubMed]
6. Saluja, G.; Brenner, R.; Morrongiello, B.A.; Haynie, D.; Rivera, M.; Cheng, T.L. The role of supervision in child injury risk: Definition, conceptual and measurement issues. *Inj. Control Saf. Promot.* **2004**, *11*, 17–22. [CrossRef] [PubMed]
7. Peterson, L.; Ewigman, B.; Kivlahan, C. Judgments regarding appropriate child supervision to prevent injury: The role of environmental risk and child age. *Child Dev.* **1993**, *64*, 934–950. [CrossRef] [PubMed]
8. Morrongiello, B.A.; Kiriakou, S. Mother' home-safety practices for preventing six types of childhood injuries: What do they do, and why? *J. Pediatr. Psychol.* **2004**, *29*, 285–297. [CrossRef] [PubMed]
9. Wills, K.E.; Christoffel, K.K.; Lavigne, J.V.; Tanz, R.R.; Schofer, J.L.; Donovan, M.; Kalangis, K. Patterns and correlates of supervision in child pedestrian injury. The Kids "N" Cars Research Team. *J. Pediatr. Psychol.* **1997**, *22*, 89–104. [CrossRef] [PubMed]
10. Blum, C.; Shield, J. Toddler drowning in domestic swimming pools. *Inj. Prev.* **2000**, *6*, 288–290. [CrossRef] [PubMed]
11. Bugeja, L.; Franklin, R. Drowning deaths of zero- to five-year-old children in Victorian dams, 1989–2001. *Aust. J. Rural Health* **2005**, *13*, 300–308. [CrossRef] [PubMed]
12. Cass, D.T.; Ross, F.; Lam, L.T. Childhood drowning in New South Wales 1990–1995: A population-based study. *Med. J. Aust.* **1996**, *165*, 610–612. [PubMed]
13. Jensen, L.R.; Williams, S.D.; Thurman, D.J.; Keller, P.A. Submersion injuries in children younger than 5 years in urban Utah. *West. J. Med.* **1992**, *157*, 641–644. [PubMed]
14. Kemp, A.M.; Mott, A.M.; Sibert, J.R. Accidents and child abuse in bathtub submersions. *Arch. Dis. Child.* **1994**, *70*, 435–438. [CrossRef] [PubMed]
15. Rauchschwalbe, R.; Brenner, R.A.; Smith, G.S. The role of bathtub seats and rings in infant drowning deaths. *Pediatrics* **1997**, *100*, E1. [CrossRef] [PubMed]
16. Ross, F.I.; Elliott, E.J.; Lam, L.T.; Cass, D.T. Children under 5 years presenting to paediatricians with near-drowning. *J. Paediatr. Child Health* **2003**, *39*, 446–450. [CrossRef] [PubMed]
17. Simon, H.K.; Tamura, T.; Colton, K. Reported level of supervision of young children while in the bathtub. *Ambul. Pediatr.* **2003**, *3*, 106–108. [CrossRef]
18. Somers, G.R.; Chiasson, D.A.; Smith, C.R. Pediatric drowning: A 20-year review of autopsied cases: III. Bathtub drownings. *Am. J. Forensic Med. Pathol.* **2006**, *27*, 113–116. [CrossRef] [PubMed]
19. Kemp, A.; Sibert, J.R. Drowning and near drowning in children in the United Kingdom: Lessons for prevention. *BMJ* **1992**, *304*, 1143–1146. [CrossRef] [PubMed]
20. Hyder, A.A.; Alonge, O.; He, S.; Wadhwaniya, S.; Rahman, F.; Rahman, A.; Arifeen, S.E. Saving of children's lives from drowning project in Bangladesh. *Am. J. Prev. Med.* **2014**, *47*, 842–845. [CrossRef] [PubMed]
21. Rahman, A.F.R.; Shafinaz, S.; Linnan, M. *Bangladesh Health and Injury Survey: Report on Children*; UNICEF: Dhaka, Bangladesh, 2005; pp. 1–202.
22. Leavy, J.E.; Crawford, G.; Franklin, R.; Denehy, M.; Jancey, J.D. Drowning. In *The International Encyclopedia of Public Health*, 2nd ed.; Quah, S.R., Ed.; Oliver Walter: Waltham, MA, USA, 2017; Volume 2, pp. 361–365.
23. Petrass, L.; Blitvich, J.D.; Finch, C.F. Parent/caregiver supervision and child injury: A systematic review of critical dimensions for understanding this relationship. *Fam. Community Health* **2009**, *32*, 123–135. [CrossRef] [PubMed]
24. Morrongiello, B.A.; Pickett, W.; Berg, R.L.; Linneman, J.G.; Brison, R.J.; Marlenga, B. Adult supervision and pediatric injuries in the agricultural worksite. *Accid. Anal. Prev.* **2008**, *40*, 1149–1156. [CrossRef] [PubMed]
25. Morrongiello, B.A.; McArthur, B.A. Parent supervision to prevent injuries. In *Encyclopedia of Early Childhood Development*, 2nd ed.; Tremblay, R.E., Ed.; University of Guelph: Guelph, ON, Canada, 2014; pp. 1–6.
26. Morrongiello, B.A.; Schell, S.L.; Schmidt, S. "Please keep an eye on your younger sister": Sibling supervision and young children's risk of unintentional injury. *Inj. Prev.* **2010**, *16*, 398–402. [CrossRef] [PubMed]

27. Holder, Y.; Peden, M.; Krug, E.; Lund, J.; Gururaj, G.; Kobusingye, O. (Eds.) *Injury Surveillance Guidelines*; World Health Organization: Geneva, Switzerland, 2001; pp. 1–80. Available online: http://apps.who.int/iris/handle/10665/42451 (accessed on 5 April 2017).
28. Ramp, B.A.; Van't Klooster, M.; de Hoog, M.; Jansen, N.J.; Oudesluys-Murphy, H.M. Childhood drowning in The Netherlands. *Nederlands Tijdschrift Voor Geneeskunde* **2014**, *158*, A7396. [PubMed]
29. Bamber, A.R.; Pryce, J.W.; Ashworth, M.T.; Sebire, N.J. Immersion-related deaths in infants and children: Autopsy experience from a specialist center. *Forensic Sci. Med. Pathol.* **2014**, *10*, 363–370. [CrossRef] [PubMed]
30. Thompson, D.C.; Rivara, F.P. Pool fencing for preventing drowning in children. *Cochrane Database Syst. Rev.* **1998**. [CrossRef]
31. Wallis, B.A.; Watt, K.; Franklin, R.C.; Taylor, M.; Nixon, J.W.; Kimble, R.M. Interventions associated with drowning prevention in children and adolescents: Systematic literature review. *Inj. Prev.* **2015**, *21*, 195–204. [CrossRef] [PubMed]
32. Leavy, J.E.; Crawford, G.; Leaversuch, F.; Nimmo, L.; McCausland, K.; Jancey, J. A review of drowning prevention interventions for children and young people in high, low and middle income countries. *J. Community Health* **2016**, *41*, 424–441. [CrossRef] [PubMed]
33. Committee on Injury, Violence, and Poison Prevention. Prevention of drowning in infants, children, and adolescents. *Pediatrics* **2003**, *112*, 437–439. Available online: http://www.ncbi.nlm.nih.gov/pubmed/12897305 (accessed on 14 September 2016).
34. Brenner, R.A. Prevention of drowning in infants, children, and adolescents. *Pediatrics* **2003**, *112*, 440–445. [CrossRef] [PubMed]
35. Morrongiello, B.A.; House, K. Measuring parent attributes and supervision behaviors relevant to child injury risk: Examining the usefulness of questionnaire measures. *Inj. Prev.* **2004**, *10*, 114–118. [CrossRef] [PubMed]
36. Morrongiello, B.A.; Sandomierski, M.; Spence, J.R. Changes over swim lessons in parents' perceptions of children's supervision needs in drowning risk situations: "His swimming has improved so now he can keep himself safe". *Health Psychol.* **2014**, *33*, 608–615. [CrossRef] [PubMed]
37. Guilfoyle, S.M.; Karazsia, B.T.; Langkamp, D.L.; Wildman, B.G. Supervision to prevent childhood unintentional injury: Developmental knowledge and self-efficacy count. *J. Child Health Care* **2012**, *16*, 141–152. [CrossRef] [PubMed]
38. Butler, F.R.; Zakari, N. Grandparents parenting grandchildren: Assessing health status, parental stress and social supports. *J. Gerontol. Nurs.* **2005**, *31*, 43–54. [CrossRef] [PubMed]
39. Grinstead, L.N.; Leder, S.; Jensen, S.; Bond, L. Review of research on the health of caregiving grandparents. *J. Adv. Nurs.* **2003**, *44*, 318–326. [CrossRef] [PubMed]
40. Musil, C.M.; Gordon, N.L.; Warner, C.B.; Zauszniewski, J.A.; Standing, T.; Wykle, M. Grandmothers and caregiving to grandchildren: Continuity, change, and outcomes over 24 months. *Gerontologlist* **2011**, *51*, 86–100. [CrossRef] [PubMed]
41. Bishai, D.; Trevitt, J.L.; Zhang, Y.; McKenzie, L.B.; Leventhal, T.; Gielen, A.C.; Guyer, B. Risk factors for unintentional injuries in children: Are grandparents protective? *Pediatrics* **2008**, *122*, e980–e987. [CrossRef] [PubMed]
42. Rahman, F.; Bose, S.; Linnan, M.; Rahman, A.; Mashreky, S.; Haaland, B.; Finkelstein, E. Cost-effectiveness of an injury and drowning prevention program in Bangladesh. *Pediatrics* **2012**, *130*, e1621–e1628. [CrossRef] [PubMed]
43. Phelan, K.J.; Morrongiello, B.A.; Khoury, J.C.; Xu, Y.; Liddy, S.; Lanphear, B. Maternal supervision of children during their first 3 years of life: The influence of maternal depression and child gender. *J. Pediatr. Psychol.* **2014**, *39*, 349–357. [CrossRef] [PubMed]
44. Ernster, V.L. Nested case-control studies. *Prev. Med.* **1994**, *23*, 587–590. [CrossRef] [PubMed]
45. Soori, H.; Khodakarim, S. Child unintentional injury prevention in Eastern Mediterranean Region. *Int. J. Crit. Illn. Inj. Sci.* **2016**, *6*, 33–39. [CrossRef] [PubMed]

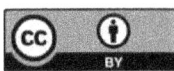

International Journal of
*Environmental Research
and Public Health*

MDPI

Article

Care-Seeking Patterns and Direct Economic Burden of Injuries in Bangladesh

Yira Natalia Alfonso [1,*], Olakunle Alonge [2], Dewan Md Emdadul Hoque [3],
Md Kamran Ul Baset [4], Adnan A. Hyder [2] and David Bishai [1]

[1]   Department of Population Family and Reproductive health, International Injury Research Unit,
      Johns Hopkins University Bloomberg School of Public Health, Baltimore, MD 21205, USA; dbishai@jhu.edu
[2]   Department of International Health, International Injury Research Unit,
      Johns Hopkins University Bloomberg School of Public Health, Baltimore, MD 21205, USA;
      oalonge1@jhu.edu (O.A.); ahyder1@jhu.edu (A.A.H.)
[3]   Maternal and Child Health Division, International Centre for Diarrhoeal Disease Research Bangladesh,
      Dhaka 1212, Bangladesh; emdad@icddrb.org
[4]   Centre for Injury Prevention and Research, Dhaka 1206, Bangladesh; kamran_baset@yahoo.co.uk
*   Correspondence: ynalfonso@jhu.edu

Academic Editor: Ulf-G. Gerdtham
Received: 6 February 2017; Accepted: 21 April 2017; Published: 29 April 2017

Abstract: This study provides a comprehensive review of the care-seeking patterns and direct economic burden of injuries from the victims' perspective in rural Bangladesh using a 2013 household survey covering 1.17 million people. Descriptive statistics and bivariate analyses were used to derive rates and test the association between variables. An analytic model was used to estimate total injury out-of-pocket (OOP) payments and a multivariate probit regression model assessed the relationship between financial distress and injury type. Results show non-fatal injuries occur to 1 in 5 people in our sample per year. With average household size of 4.5 in Bangladesh–every household has an injury every year. Most non-fatally injured patients sought healthcare from drug sellers. Less than half of fatal injuries sought healthcare and half of those with care were hospitalized. Average OOP payments varied significantly (range: $8–$830) by injury type and outcome (fatal vs. non-fatal). Total injury OOP expenditure was $355,795 and $5000 for non-fatal and fatal injuries, respectively, per 100,000 people. The majority of household heads with injuries reported financial distress. This study can inform injury prevention advocates on disparities in healthcare usage, OOP costs and financial distress. Reallocation of resources to the most at risk populations can accelerate reduction of preventable injuries and prevent injury related catastrophic payments and impoverishment.

Keywords: injuries; cost; out-of-pocket; economic burden; care-seeking patterns; low-and-middle-income countries; Bangladesh

---

1. Introduction

In Bangladesh, the burden of disease from injuries in 2013 was 3031 disability-adjusted-life-years (DALYs) per 100,000 people, which was slightly lower than the global rate, 3456 DALYs per 100,000, and made about 10% of the national disease burden [1]. To prevent injury related disabilities and deaths prompt access to high quality post-injury healthcare is crucial. However, there is increasing evidence across low-and-middle-income-countries (LMIC) that there are major barriers to access health facilities and surgical care [2]. Some of these barriers include long distance to facilities, poor roads and lack of suitable transport, few healthcare providers with resources and expertise, fear of healthcare procedures, high direct and indirect costs related to healthcare as well as socioeconomic status [2]. Barriers to access perpetuate patients' preferences for self-care, faith on traditional healers (e.g., consultation with

Kabiraji/hakimiand homeopathic practitioners), unqualified allopathic providers or para-professionals (village practitioners with a year-long training) [3], and may also reduce completion of healthcare treatments. Further, either high healthcare expenditures or inadequately treated injuries that reduce individual's work productivity can push families into financial distress (i.e., reduce household income or assets to pay for basic necessities such as food, clothing, housing, school, etc.) worsening the burden from injuries.

Out of the total health expenditure of $16.20 per capita in 2010, 64% was covered out-of-pocket (OOP), 26% by public funds and the remaining by international development partners [4,5]. Between 1997–2007 OOP grew at 14% annually, faster than the annual gross domestic product (GDP), 10% [5]. Similarly, a cross-sectional study from 2009 showed that 94% of injury victims in Bangladesh had an OOP expenditure related to the injury [6]. The growing reliance on OOP expenditures to cover healthcare costs places a large economic burden on individuals needing healthcare services.

When injury related healthcare costs are high compared to family income, payments can absorb a large fraction of household resources resulting in catastrophic expenditures. Injury related expenditures can result from direct medical costs (hospitalization, medicines, labs, etc.), direct non-medical (transportation, food, and accommodation, funeral), indirect costs (income loss due to disability or for caring for a family member with disability), or non-monetary/intangible costs (of premature death, pain and suffering, etc.) [7]. Many south Asian countries like Bangladesh and India have high prevalence of catastrophic payments related to injuries [8–10].

This study uses 2013 data from a household survey in rural Bangladesh to better understand care-seeking patterns for injuries and the economic burden on victims. The specific aims of this study were to describe care-seeking patterns by injury type, demographic and socioeconomic characteristics; to evaluate injuries' OOP expenditures by injury type and type of cost; and assess the extent of financial distress due to injury related expenditures. Given the data available, this study evaluates the direct economic burden of injuries from the perspective of the injury victim during the short-term and excludes indirect costs.

2. Methods

The data used is from a household survey covering 51 unions (the smallest rural administrative and local government units) from seven sub-districts in rural Bangladesh and was comparable to the 2011 Bangladesh national census [11]. The survey was conducted over a 6-month period (June–November 2013) and covered all 1.17 million individuals in these unions. The survey collected data for all members of a household. Details on the household survey objectives, population, sample design and data management are provided elsewhere [12,13]. This survey was part of the data collected for the Saving of Lives from Drowning (SoLiD) intervention [14,15]. Given that the survey's recall period for non-fatal injuries was 6 months and for fatal injuries was 1 year, we multiply rates for injuries and cost data for non-fatal injuries by two in order to present all results in person-year units.

Descriptive statistics were used to estimate injury rates and the proportion of each injury out of all injuries by sex, age group and SES (socioeconomic status). Similarly, descriptive statistics were used to estimate the percent of injured persons seeking healthcare by injury type, type of healthcare provider, type of health facility or treatment site, the median number of hospitalization days, and health outcomes (recovered, improving and no improvement). The Chi-squared statistical test was used to assess the association between care provider and injury type as well as, for those hospitalized, injury type and health outcome [16].

Descriptive statistics were also used to estimate the proportion of injured individuals with OOP payments greater than zero and the average expenditure among individuals with payments greater than zero by injury type and type of cost (e.g., consultation cost, laboratory cost, bed cost, operation cost, medicine cost, attendant cost, transportation cost, other cost, and total cost). The overall average spending is defined as:

$$\text{Average Spending} = \text{Pr.(Spend} > 0) \times \text{E(Spend | Spend} > 0) \tag{1}$$

Expenditure data was inflation adjusted from 2013 to 2016 Bangladeshi Taka using inflation index 1.21437 and currency converted to 2016 U.S. dollars using conversion rate of 0.0152. The Wilcoxon-Mann-Whitney statistical test, a non-parametric analog to the independent samples t-test, was used to assess the association between injury type or the probability of getting treatment and OOP expenditures [17,18]. A decision analytic model was developed estimating the total per injury cost for every 100,000 people [7]. This model multiplied the probability of each type of event by the cost of each event.

Care-seeking patterns and OOP cost estimates were derived separately for non-fatal (injury outcome reported was survived) and fatal (injury outcome reported was death) injuries.

Financial distress was assessed by first estimating the proportion of injured individuals who reported using a financial coping mechanism (e.g., borrow money from relatives/friends, reduced consumption of basic goods, reduced food consumption, took loans, sold assets, other) to cover injury related costs. Then, a probit multivariate regression analysis assessed the association between financial distress (using any financial coping mechanism) and type of injury controlling for demographic and socioeconomic characteristics [19], see Equation (2):

$$\begin{aligned} FIN\_Distress_i = \quad & \beta_0 + \beta_1 Injuries_i + \beta_2 Severity_i + \beta_3 Female_i + \beta_4 School_i \\ & + \beta_5 HHsize_i + \beta_6 Age_i + \beta_6 District_i + \beta_6 SES_i + \varepsilon_i \end{aligned} \tag{2}$$

Where *FIN_Distress* is a binomial dependent variable equal to one if the injured person used any financial coping mechanism, β_0 is the constant term, and Injuries is a vector of ten injury dummies where the base case (the least frequent injuries, which made less than 1% of the injury burden and had the lowest total OOP: drowning, suffocation, suicide attempt and unintentional poisoning) is omitted. Thus, the coefficient β_1 is interpreted as the probability of financial distress (multiplied by 100) compared to the base case, holding all other variables constant. Control variables included: Severity, a vector of three dummies where medium and high severity are compared to the omitted dummy of low severity; Female, a dummy for sex; School, a dummy for secondary education; District, a vector of place of residence including Narshindi, Camilla, and Chandpur compared to the omitted base case Sherpur/Siraigonj; SES, a vector of four socioeconomic status with the high income group as the omitted base case; and Age, a vector of four age groups with under-fifteen as the omitted base case. The marginal effect of each coefficient is estimated holding all other coefficients at the mean. The household survey only collected data on use of financial coping mechanism from the injured individuals who were a source of family income (either a minor, main, or major source of family income). Thus, the regression analysis excludes the injuries from individuals who were not contributors to the family income (i.e., children, household keepers, elders or unemployed adults). As such, these estimates likely underestimate the extent of financial distress among all families with an injured family member.

3. Results

The study included 1,169,593 individuals from 270,387 households. Details on demographic and injury rates of the study population are provided elsewhere (see Supplementary Materials) [12,13]. Annually there were 238,929 injuries during the year prior to the survey among 209,059 individuals (17.9% of the population). In other words, almost 1 out of every 5 individuals had at least one injury during the year. The total injury rate was 20,428 per 100,000 people. Among the injured, 0.2% (449) died due to the injury. Among those with non-fatal injuries, 11.5% (23,976) and 2.2% (4496) had a second and third injury, respectively. Among non-fatal injuries, only 0.3% of the injury data was missing. The non-fatal injury rate was 20,390 per 100,000 people (238,480 total injuries); falls had the highest rate (7741), followed by cuts (4499) and blunt object injuries (2015). The total fatal-injury rate was 38 per 100,000 people (449 total injuries); the highest was among drowning (15), followed by transport injuries (7) and falls (5).

3.1. Healthcare Seeking Patterns and Hospitalization

Overall, 88% of the non-fatal injured sought healthcare treatment; 80% went to a pharmacy/medicine shop, 81% got care from a drug seller/village doctors and 3% were hospitalized (Table 1). The probability of care was not largely different between low, medium and high injury severity levels, ranging from 85% to 94% (see Supplementary Materials). Out of those hospitalized, 34% recovered and 62% were still improving at the time of the survey. Suicides (36%) and poisoning injuries (24%) were most likely to be hospitalized. Among the fatally injured, 45% sought treatment; among the treated, 67% and 48% of healthcare was provided by a doctor and at a hospital, respectively, and 51% were hospitalized.

Table 1. Annual care-seeking patterns, hospitalization and health outcome rates of injured persons

Injury Care-Seeking Patterns (Percent Values Are × 100)	Non-Fatal Injuries	Fatal Injuries
Annual number of injuries	238,480	449
Percent that sought treatment	0.88	0.45
Out of the total with treatment, percent that received healthcare from each type of provider		
Drug seller/Village doctor	0.81	0.21
Registered doctor	0.14	0.67
Traditional healer/Religious Leader	0.06	0.07
Medical Assistant/SACMO	0.03	0.22
HA/FWV/FWA	0.01	0.02
Other (NGO, homeopathic practitioner, trained TBA)	0.02	0.03
Out of the total with treatment, percent that received healthcare from each type of healthcare facility		
Pharmacy/medicine shop keeper	0.8	0.16
Private (Clinic or practitioner's chamber)	0.1	0.22
Own home	0.08	0.07
Upazila Health Complex	0.04	0.25
Hospital (District or Specialized)	0.04	0.48
Clinic (NGO or Public Primary Health)	0.01	
UHFWC—Union Health and Family Welfare Centres	0.01	0.04
Other	0.02	
Hospitalization among those treated		
Hospitalizations	0.03	0.51
Median number of hospitalization days	4	4
Treatment outcome among those with hospitalizations		
Recovered	0.34	-
Improving	0.62	-
No improvement	0.04	-

Sub-Assistant Community Medical Officer (SACMO); Health Assistant (HA); Family Welfare Visitor (FWV) or Assistant (FWA). Details on care-seeking patterns by injury type are provided in the Supplementary Materials.

3.2. Out-of-Pocket Expenditures Related to Injury Treatment

The majority of non-fatal injuries (96%) reported an OOP expense. The Mann-Whitney statistic showed a statistically significant association between OOP costs and getting treatment as well as getting treatment from a registered doctor (*p*-value 0.000). The total annual non-fatal OOP expenditure was $4.16 million (a rate of $355,795 per every 100,000 people) and the average OOP cost (excluding the 4% of injuries with zero expenditure) was $21. The probability of expenditures between the lowest and highest SES only varied from 95% to 97%. Among those with expenditures, the mean expenditure between SES levels varied from between $16 and $26 for the low and high SES groups respectively. Out of the total expenditure, the majority is from falls (43%) and transport injuries (22%) (see Figure 1a). The highest average OOP costs were for suicide attempt ($84), unintentional poisoning ($55), violence ($47) and transport ($46) (see Figure 2a). The probability of OOP payments for medicines was 95%, for transport 31% and for consultation fees 15%. Medicines made 65% of the total OOP cost. Details on costs by injury type and cost category are provided in the Supplementary Materials.

Among fatal injuries, 74% incurred OOP expenses. The total fatal-injury OOP expenditure was $59,672 (a rate of $5114 per 100,000 people) and the average (excluding the 26% of injuries with zero expenditure) was $395 (see Supplementary Materials). Out of the total cost, the majority is from transport injuries (33%), falls (22%), and burn injuries (22%) (see Figure 1b). The highest average OOP costs among fatal injuries were due to machine injuries ($830), transport ($760), cuts ($710) and burns ($704). Similarly, the average cost was highest for surgeries, followed by medicines, and hospital beds (see Supplementary Materials). The average expenditure, for injuries with expenses greater than zero, was 38% of the total GDPpc ($1033) and for the more costly injuries was between 68% (burns) to 80% (machine injuries) of the GDPpc [20].

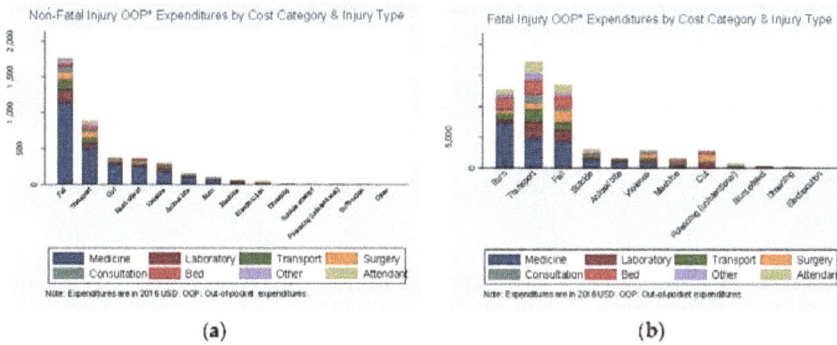

Figure 1. Total direct out-of-pocket expenditure from injuries for every 100,000 people from the study area.

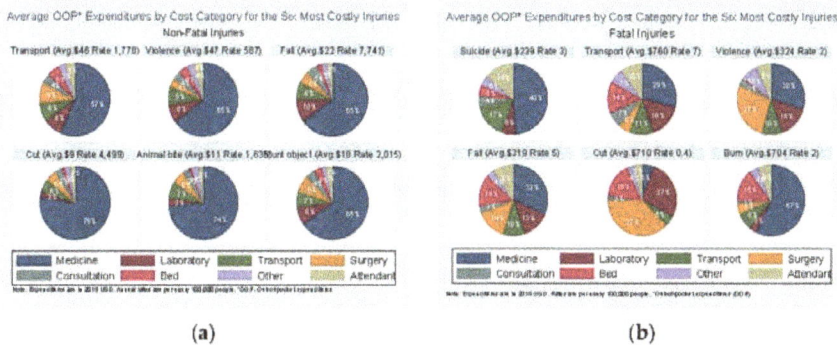

Figure 2. Non-fatal injuries direct average cost by cost category and injury type.

3.3. Financial Coping Mechanisms

Among the individuals with non-fatal and fatal injuries, 35% and 27%, respectively, were a source of family income. Most of these individuals were married males, a third had secondary education and 95% where over eighteen years old. Among this group, 90% reported using at least one financial coping mechanism to cover injury related costs. Borrowing money was the most frequent mechanism and more prevalent among fatal injuries than non-fatal injuries (56% vs. 29%). In bivariate analysis, the probability of financial distress was not statistically different by type of injury (see Supplementary Materials). Similarly, multivariate regression analysis, controlling for all injury types, demographic and SES factors, showed no association between financial distress and injury type, expect for a slight positive association between violence or machine injuries (2.8% or 3.3% respectively, p-value < 0.05) and financial distress compared to the base case (see Table 2).

Table 2. Regression results on association between financial distress and injury type.

Variables	1	2	3	4	5
	Fin. Stress	Fin. Stress	Fin. Stress	Fin. Stress	Fin. Stress
Injury: Transport	0.023 *	0.020	0.017	0.017	0.018
Injury: Violence	0.037 ***	0.033 **	0.031 **	0.029 **	0.028 **
Injury: Fall	0.025 **	0.024 **	0.026 **	0.018	0.018
Injury: Cut	0.012	0.015	0.015	0.018	0.018
Injury: Burn	0.001	0.005	0.010	0.015	0.016
Injury: Machine	0.038 ***	0.038 ***	0.034**	0.032 **	0.033 **
Injury: Electrocution	0.007	0.008	0.007	0.009	0.010
Injury: Animal Bite	0.000	0.005	0.006	0.009	0.010
Injury: Blunt Object	0.012	0.021 *	0.019	0.013	0.013
Injury severity: Medium		0.031 ***	0.03 ***	0.022 ***	0.022 ***
Injury severity: High		0.022 ***	0.021 ***	0.016 ***	0.016 ***
Family/household size			0.002 ***	0.001 **	0.001 **
Female			−0.014 ***	−0.006 ***	−0.006 ***
Secondary education			0.005 **	0.001	0.002
Age: 15–24 yrs.				0.006	0.005
Age: 25–64 yrs.				0.01 **	0.01 **
Age: 65+ yrs.				0.013 **	0.013 ***
District: Chandpur				0.053 ***	0.053 ***
District: Sherpur				−0.011 ***	−0.011 ***
District: Narshindi				−0.010 ***	−0.010 ***
SES: Medium					0.006 **
SES: Low					0.008 ***
SES: Lowest					0.006 **
Observations	42,327	42,327	42,327	42,327	42,327

*** $p < 0.01$, ** $p < 0.05$, * $p < 0.1$. Data includes the injuries from individuals who were a source of family income (35% of total fatal-injuries). Data excludes fatal injuries. Coefficients are interpreted as percentage point changes × 100 compared to their base case. The base case are the least frequent injuries with lowest total OOP: suffocation, suicide attempt, poisoning and drowning. For example, among this sub-set of the population, there is a 2.8% percentage point increase in the probability of financial distress among violence injuries compared to the base case, holding other factors constant. For details and regression tests see the Supplementary Materials.

4. Discussion

This study evaluated the care-seeking patterns and economic burden of injured individuals in Bangladesh using a household survey from 2013 covering 1.17 million rural people. Overall, non-fatal injuries occur to 1 in 5 people in our sample per year. With average household size of 4.5 in Bangladesh—every household has an injury every year. Highest risk age group is 25 to 64 year olds followed by 5 to 9 year olds. Risk is 1.3 times higher in males than females. Care-seeking patterns show that the probability of seeking treatment is lower for non-fatal than fatal injuries (88% vs. 45% respectively). Among non-fatal injuries, most individuals sought healthcare services from drug sellers/village doctors and at a pharmacy shop. A similar study on burn injuries among 0–18 year olds also found that a significant portion sought care from unqualified service providers (60% vs. 85%

and 17% from non- and fatal injuries, respectively) [21]. Among the fatally injured individuals that sought treatment, less than half received care at a hospital.

Almost all (96%) of non-fatal injuries require out of pocket costs and average $21 and $395 (which is 38% of the Bangladeshi gross domestic product (GDP) per capita, $1033 in 2013) for non- and fatal injuries, respectively. A third of the OOP cost was from medicine expenditures, averaging $13 and $178 for non- and fatal injuries respectively. The low probability for seeking registered doctors and hospitalization may be explained by barriers to healthcare access or OOP costs deterring usage [2,9]. For instance, among non-fatal injuries with OOP expenditures, the average cost for care by a registered doctor was $76 higher than by other healthcare providers, or getting care at a hospital or clinic was $69 higher than getting care at a pharmacy or home. Similarly, among fatal injuries, being hospitalized cost on average $545 more than not being hospitalized. These large direct OOP payments are catastrophic expenditures and can push households into poverty.

The largest portion of OOP expenditure was from falls and transport injures. These injuries were among the costliest because of their high injury rate and average cost. Transport injuries had a hospitalization rate of 7% with a median of 3 hospitalization days. A similar study on transport injuries in Bangladesh found that these injuries were responsible for 5% of hospitalizations in primary and secondary level hospitals, averaged 5.7 hospitalized days and cost on average $86 (in 2010 USD) [22]. Another study on burn injuries found an average cost of $217 (in 2008 USD) compared to $11 and $704 for non- and fatal injuries, respectively, in this study [23]. Drowning, suffocation and electrocution had the lowest average cost because these were the least likely to seek care. But, if indirect costs were included, these fatal injuries would be the costliest due to their lifelong lost productivity/income.

Previous evidence also showed that the majority of injured victims in Bangladesh had OOP expenditures and similarly mostly for medicines, but average medicine OOP cost were lower than in this study ($4 vs. $13) [6]. While this value may seem a small fraction out of the total GDP per capita, this cost can be catastrophic for families in rural areas which has reported suffering from a 36% poverty rate, inadequate diet, periods of food shortage, and having half of the children chronically malnourished [24]. Similarly, among fatal injuries, the average direct OOP cost is 38% of the GDP per capita.

Reducing the direct economic burden of injured individuals could save Bangladesh $356 thousand plus $5 thousand, from non-fatal and fatal injuries, respectively, for every 100,000 people. These costs only reflect short-term direct savings but are substantially higher if considering the long-term direct OOP costs and indirect costs. Prior evidence from LMICs show that while the median direct medical cost for hospitalization was $291 (range $14–17,400), after adding indirect costs, the median cost increased a 14-fold to US$4085 (range: $17–10,300) or 97% of GDP per capita [25]. While the indirect cost and long-term direct estimates are beyond the scoop of this study, this study's results show that most household heads with injuries suffered financial distress from injury treatment related costs.

This study was limited by six months (for non-fatal injuries) to one year (for fatal injuries) of self-reported injury and healthcare use and cost data. Also results only captured the short-term effects of injuries. A longer study period could capture the long-term direct costs, particularly for the majority of injuries still in recovery (64%) at the time of the survey. This study also excludes the economic burden from indirect costs which are higher than direct costs [26,27]. Similarly, direct medical costs covered by other public and private financing sources are not included. However, this study's focus was on capturing the direct OOP expenditures which are often not available in the cost of healthcare studies. Lastly, financial coping mechanisms data was only available for the sub-group of the population with injuries who were a source of family income. Data on financial coping mechanisms from all injured individuals would show the full extent of financial distress among families with injured members.

5. Conclusions

Non-fatal injuries occur to 1 in 5 people in our sample per year. Living in Bangladesh imposes an "injury tax" of $21 per household per year. This does not account for indirect costs, the pain, suffering, and income losses. High risk makes this a prevalent pathway into economic distress. One of the best things Bangladesh can do for its citizens and its economy is to make communities safer. There are promising policies that Bangladeshi communities can use to remove this "injury tax". Leading economic risks are falls, transport, cuts, blunt objects, violence, animal bites, and burns. Measures include enforce occupational safety regulations, worksite inspection, home safety inspection and promotion, CHW (community health worker) training on safe homes and farms, animal control for stray/wild dogs.

Supplementary Materials: The following are available online at http://www.mdpi.com/1660-4601/14/5/472/s1, Care-Seeking Patterns and Direct Economic Burden of Injuries in Bangladesh.

Acknowledgments: This research was funded by Bloomberg Philanthropies.

Author Contributions: Yira Natalia Alfonso conceptualized the idea, conducted the analysis, wrote the first draft and managed revisions. David Bishai conceptualized the idea, revised the analysis and edited the manuscript. Olakunle Alonge, Adnan A. Hyder, Dewan Md Emdadul Hoque, and Md Kamran Ul Baset conceptualized the idea, managed the data collection and reviewed the manuscript.

Conflicts of Interest: The authors declare no conflict of interest.

Abbreviations

The following abbreviations are used in this manuscript:

OOP	Out-of-pocket
LMIC	Low-and-middle-income-countries
HIC	High-income-countries
NGO	Non-governmental organization
SES	Socioeconomic status
GDP	Gross domestic product

References

1. Institute for Health Metrics and Evaluation (IHME). GBD Compare—GBD Super Regions Pyramid. Available online: http://vizhub.healthdata.org/gbd-compare (accessed on 10 June 2016).
2. Grimes, C.E.; Bowman, K.G.; Dodgion, C.M.; Lavy, C.B.D. Systematic review of barriers to surgical care in low-income and middle-income countries. *World J. Surgery* **2011**, *35*, 941–950. [CrossRef] [PubMed]
3. Ahmed, S.M.; Adams, A.M.; Chowdhury, M.; Bhuiya, A. Changing health-seeking behaviour in matlab, Bangladesh: Do development interventions matter? *Health Policy Plan.* **2003**, *18*, 306–315. [CrossRef]
4. Islam, A.; Biswas, T. Health system in Bangladesh: Challenges and opportunities. *Am. J. Health Res.* **2014**, *2*, 366–374. [CrossRef]
5. Ahmed, S.M.; Alam, B.; Anwar, I.; Begun, T.; Huque, R.; Khan, J.; Nababan, H.; Osman, F. *Bangladesh Health System Review*; Asia Pacific Observatory on Health Systems and Policies: New Delhi, India, 2015.
6. Dalal, K.; Rahman, A. Out-of-pocket payments for unintentional injuries: A study in rural Bangladesh. *Intern. J. Inj. Contr. Saf. Promot.* **2009**, *16*, 41–47. [CrossRef] [PubMed]
7. Drummond, M.F.; Sculpher, M.J.; Claxton, K.; Stoddart, G.L.; Torrance, G.W. *Methods for the Economic Evaluation of Health Care Programmes*; Oxford University Press: London, UK, 2005.
8. O'Donnell, O.; van Doorslaer, E.; Rannan-Eliya, R.P.; Somanathan, A.; Adhikari, S.R.; Akkazieva, B.; Harbianto, D.; Garg, C.C.; Hanvoravongchai, P.; Herrin, A.N.; et al. Who pays for health care in Asia? *J. Health Econ.* **2008**, *27*, 460–475.
9. Van Doorslaer, E.; O'Donnell, O.; Rannan-Eliya, R. *Paying Out-of-Pocket for Health Care in Asia: Catastrophic and poverty Impact*; Erasmus University Rotterdam: Colombo, Sri Lanka, 2005.
10. Van Doorslaer, E.; O'Donnell, O.; Rannan-Eliya, R.P.; Somanathan, A.; Adhikari, S.R.; Garg, C.C.; Harbianto, D.; Herrin, A.N.; Huq, M.N.; Ibragimova, S.; et al. Catastrophic payments for health care in Asia. *Health Econ.* **2007**, *16*, 1159–1184. [CrossRef] [PubMed]
11. Bangladesh Bureau of Statistics (BBS). 2011 Population and Housing Census. Available online: http://203.112.218.65/Census.aspx?MenuKey=43 (accessed on 10 June 2016).

12. Alonge, O.; Agrawal, P.; Talab, A.; Rahman, Q.; Rahman, F.; Arifeen, S.; Hyder, A. Fatal and non-fatal injury outcomes in Bangladesh: Results from a large population study. *Lancet* **2017**, under review.

13. He, S.; Alonge, O.; Agrawal, P.; Sharmin, S.; Islam, I.; Mashreky, S.; Arifeen, S. Epidemiology of burns in rural Bangladesh: An update. *Int. J. Environ. Res. Public Health* **2017**, *14*, 381. [CrossRef] [PubMed]

14. Hyder, A.A.; Alonge, O.; He, S.; Wadhwaniya, S.; Rahman, F.; Rahman, A.; Arifeen, S.E. Saving of children's lives from drowning project in Bangladesh. *Am. J. Prev. Med.* **2014**, *47*, 842–845. [CrossRef] [PubMed]

15. Hyder, A.A.; Alonge, O.; He, S.; Wadhwaniya, S.; Rahman, F.; Rahman, A.; Arifeen, S.E. A framework for addressing implementation gap in global drowning prevention interventions: Experiences from Bangladesh. *J. Health Popul. Nutr.* **2014**, *32*, 564–576.

16. Rao, J.N.K.; Scott, A.J. The analysis of categorical data from complex sample surveys: Chi-squared tests for goodness of fit and independence in two-way tables. *J. Am. Stat. Assoc.* **1981**, *76*, 221–230. [CrossRef]

17. Wilcoxon, F. Individual comparisons by ranking methods. *Biometrics* **1945**, *1*, 80–83. [CrossRef]

18. Mann, H.B.; Whitney, D.R. On a test of whether one of two random variables is stochastically larger than the other. *Ann Math. Stat.* **1947**, *18*, 50–60. [CrossRef]

19. Aldrich, J.H.; Nelson, F.D. *The Method of Probits*; SAGE: Newbury Park, CA, USA, 1984.

20. International Monetary Fund (IMF). World Economic Outlook Database, April 2015. Available online: http://www.imf.org/external/ns/cs.aspx?id=28 (accessed on 15 November 2015).

21. Mashreky, S.R.; Rahman, A.; Chowdhury, S.M.; Svanström, L.; Shafinaz, S.; Khan, T.F.; Rahman, F. Health seeking behaviour of parents of burned children in Bangladesh is related to family socioeconomics. *Injury* **2010**, *41*, 528–532. [CrossRef] [PubMed]

22. Mashreky, S.R.; Rahman, A.; Khan, T.F.; Faruque, M.; Svanström, L.; Rahman, F. Hospital burden of road traffic injury: Major concern in primary and secondary level hospitals in Bangladesh. *Public Health* **2010**, *124*, 185–189. [CrossRef] [PubMed]

23. Mashreky, S.R.; Rahman, A.; Chowdhury, S.M.; Giashuddin, S.; Svanström, L.; Khan, T.F.; Cox, R.; Rahman, F. Burn injury: Economic and social impact on a family. *Public Health* **2008**, *122*, 1418–1424. [CrossRef] [PubMed]

24. Rural Poverty Portal. Rural Poverty in Bangladesh. Available online: http://www.ruralpovertyportal.org/country/home/tags/bangladesh# (accessed on 10 June 2016).

25. Wesson, H.K.H.; Boikhutso, N.; Bachani, A.M.; Hofman, K.J.; Hyder, A.A. The cost of injury and trauma care in low- and middle-income countries: A review of economic evidence. *Health Policy Plann.* **2014**, *29*, 795–808. [CrossRef] [PubMed]

26. Chandran, A.; Hyder, A.A.; Peek-Asa, C. The global burden of unintentional injuries and an agenda for progress. *Epidemiol Rev.* **2010**, *32*, 110–120. [CrossRef] [PubMed]

27. National Center for Injury Prevention and Control (CDC). Drowning Fatal Injuries, Nonfatal Hospitalized Injuries and Nonfatal Emergency Department Treated and Released Injuries: Both Sexes, Ages 0 to 4, United States, 2010. Available online: http://www.cdc.gov/injury/wisqars/index.html (accessed on 10 June 2016).

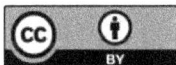

MDPI

St. Alban-Anlage 66

4052 Basel, Switzerland

Tel. +41 61 683 77 34

Fax +41 61 302 89 18

http://www.mdpi.com

International Journal of Environmental Research and Public Health Editorial
Office E-mail: ijerph@mdpi.com
http://www.mdpi.com/journal/ijerph

www.ingramcontent.com/pod-product-compliance
Lightning Source LLC
Chambersburg PA
CBHW051913210326
41597CB00033B/6127